Fortschritte der Onkologie · Band 16

Ferenc Bánhidy · Miklós Kásler

The Use of Lasers in Otorhinolaryngology and Head and Neck Surgery

Herausgegeben am Zentralinstitut für Krebsforschung
der Akademie der Wissenschaften der DDR, Berlin-Buch
von
S. Eckhardt, Budapest; St. Tanneberger, Berlin-Buch;
H. Wrba, Wien

AKADEMIE-VERLAG BERLIN

1989

Ferenc Bánhidy, MD, Professor of Head and Neck Surgery
Clinic of Head and Neck Surgery,
Postgraduate University School
of Medicine,
Budapest, Hungary

Miklós Kásler, MD, Head of Department of Head and Neck
Surgery,
National Institute of Oncology,
Budapest, Hungary

English translation: Zsófia Schoket, B. C.

ISBN 3-05-500572-4
ISSN 0323-5084
Erschienen im Akademie-Verlag Berlin, Leipziger Straße 3—4, Berlin, DDR-1086

Lizenznummer: 202 · 100/496/89
Printed in the German Democratic Republic
Gesamtherstellung: VEB Druckhaus „Maxim Gorki“, 7400 Altenburg
Lektor: Christiane Grunow
Einband: Rolf Kunze
LSV 2715
Bestellnummer: 7638829 (2165/16)
03200

Preface

The recent technical revolution has considerably changed our life and made it in all spheres most comfortable. This industrial development, however, has such drawbacks – e.g. the armament race, environmental pollution, the use of carcinogenic substances, etc. – that can hardly be controlled even by the most up-to-date means.

A peculiar product of this two-faced progress is the medical application of laser developed in the war industry.

The importance of the laser in medicine is owing to the fact that it is applicable also in those groups of diseases which are hardly curable by any effective means available, which often have a fatal outcome and where the mode of death is extremely cruel. This explains the hope and expectations towards any new procedure in the treatment of malignant tumours. The introduction of new medical techniques are preceded by a great many experiments that are gradually followed by the human application.

When writing this book we regarded it as important – in addition to describing the initial steps of the clinical use – to summarize the most significant research results because the medical application of the laser is not definitely elaborated. There are a lot of questions unanswered as yet, but the knowledge of the recent trends of investigations and their results may be highly helpful.

We express our thanks to the Academy of Sciences of the GDR for the invitation to write this book and to all those who have contributed to its publication.

The Authors

Contents

Introduction

In the field of health service series of new industrial technologies are introduced every year. The transistor pacemaker, the silastic articular prosthesis, the gamma beam sterilizer, etc. are just a few examples.

In the last decades the rapid development of the laser brought more and more up-to-date instruments into trade. These instruments provoked daring ideas in the medical practice and doctors began to believe that the laser would dominate the future and would get the victory over cancer.

The human introduction of the new procedure was carried out almost parallel to the animal experiments. It seemed to be safe since the laser has an easily controllable effect. The investigations are still under way and the doctors do not have a common stand yet. Consequently, when compiling this book we primarily aimed at discussing the possibilities of the surgical application and the widely controversial experiences. Therefore, this book is not a definitive evaluation but an introduction into the laser surgery.

Prior to describing the details it is sensible to summarize the physical principles of laser and those biological changes that can favourably affect the living tissues. The preferable indications of laser surgery are based on these biological-biochemical effects.

1. Historical Review

1.1. The major steps of research

1830 Herschel discovers the infrared ray in the spectrum of the Sun.
1831 Faraday discovers the electromagnetic induction.
1845 Faraday describes the magnetooptic phenomenon.
1862 Maxwell publishes his equations.
1875 Kerr desribes the electrooptic "Kerr-effect".
1886 Hertz – Transmission of the electromagnetic waves.
1887 Hertz is the first to observe the photo-electric effect.
1900 Planck describes the quantum theory.
1905 Einstein puts forward the hypothesis of light quantum.
1911 Rutherford creates the nucleic model named after him.
1917 Einstein – A molecule (resonator) in the radiation field may not only absorb but emit energy as well ("negative absorption", induced emission).
1919 Sommerfeld – The first review of nuclear physics.
1927 Heisenberg – The principle of uncertainty.
1928 Grotrian – The first experimental proof of induced emission.
1948 Gábor attempts to improve the resolution of the electron microscope by a two-step procedure: 1) electronic analysis, 2) optical synthesis. Establishment of holography.

1.2. The maser

After the second world war the microwave technique reached a highly advanced level. It was at this time that after Lengyel (1946) several researchers directed their investigations to the amplification of microwaves by stimulated emission (maser). Important findings are published on this subject.

1951 Purcell and Pound can detect inversion in magnetic field by a lithium-fluoride crystal.
1953 Weber – The microwaves can be amplified provided that more oscillators are in excited than in low-energy state.
1954 Gordon, Zeiger and Twones report on the first maser. When injecting the beam of stimulated ammonia molecules the emission results in a coherent radiation.
1955 Basov and Prokhorov investigate the three-level system of gas masers.
1956 Independently of Soviet scientists Bloembergen also works on a three-level solid maser system.
1957 Feher, Gordon, Buehler, Gere and Thurmond – The first pulsed solid body permaseroscillator in the two-level system.
1958 Basov, Bul and Popov, Patens – maser production by semiconductors.
1959 Javan and Saunders recommend to produce the inversion by electron impulses in a gas-discharge (mixture of neon and helium).

1.3. The laser

1960 RAUTIAN and SOBELMAN want to produce maser activity in the optic spectrum by mixing the vapour of sodium and mercury as well as by exciting a mercury lamp ($\lambda = 253.7$ nm).
ABLEKOV, PESIN and FABELINSKY exclude the use of mercury-zinc lamp in order to obtain inversion and radiation in the visible and infrared spectral range, through the stimulation of the mixture of atoms.
MAIMAN stimulates emission by a strong xenon flash-lamp when he irradiates a ruby crystal silvered on one end, thus obtaining red laser radiation ($\lambda = 694.3$ nm).
JAVAN, BENNETT, Jr. and HERRIOTT, in 1960, construct the first glass laser of continuous operation with a spectral emission of $\lambda = 1118$, 1153, 1160, 1199 and 1207 nm (near the infrared); the power of the strongest frequency is 15 mW. The gas discharge is maintained by a mixture of helium and neon. The helium-neon laser generally used nowadays ($\lambda = 632.8$ nm) was only invented in 1962.
SOROKIN and STEVENSON induce emission by three-valence uranyl ion embedded in calcium fluoride; this is the first four-level solid body laser.

1961 SOROKIN and STEVENSON are the first to use rare earth metals as active laser medium (two-valence Sm in CaF_2, CaF_2:Sm).
JOHNSON and NASSAU use neodymium as a substance for solid body laser. The element is embedded in calcium wolframate ($CaWO_4$:Nd).
SNITZER applies glass, his neodymium laser emits in the near infrared. Since 1964 mainly YAG has been used for bedding.
HELLWARTH wants to produce very short impulses by the rapid change of the reflectivity at the end of the resonator; primarily the electrooptical Kerr effect shoud be taken advantage of: this is the principle of quality modulation (Q-Switch).

1962 COLLINS and KISLIUK use a rotating disc as optical switch.
FRANKEN, HILL, PETERS and WEINREICH double the frequency of the ruby laser light by a quartz plate (second harmonic). It is the start of the non-linear optics.
KAISER and GARRETT invent the "two-photon absorption" by irradiating CaF_2:Eu crystal with the intensive light of a ruby laser.
PORTO and WOOD find that the ruby optical maser is an excellent source of light for stimulating Raman-spectra.
CAMPBELL, KOESTER et al. begin to apply ruby laser in ophthalmology.
WHITE and RIDGEN produce the well-known neon-line with the mixture of helium-neon (10:1) at 632.8 nm.
KOGELNIK and PATEL obtain pure frequency in the resonator (single mode operation) through three mirrors and Iris-diaphragm in a helium-neon laser.
RABINOWITH, JACOBS and GOULD produce laser activity in cesium-vapour with intensive helium-line irradiation at 388.8 nm.
RIDGEN and GORDON describe the granularity.
ECKHARDT, HELLWARTH, MCCLUG, SCHWARZ, WEINER and WOODBURG observe the stimulated Raman-scattering in organic substances.
BESSIS et al. – The first microirradiation of the cells by selective ruby laser absorption through Janus-green. By means of a microscope a hole with a diameter of about 2 µm can be burned.

1963 The first liquid laser works with a chelate of a rare earth metal ion.
LEMPICKI and SAMELSON use europium (Eu) in benzoyl acetone. The alcoholic solution of this organic metal complex of appropriate concentration emits red light only at lower temperature ($\lambda = 631.1$ and 615.0 nm).
BASOV and ORAEVSKII – Theory of thermic inversion in a gaseous system (heating, cooling); the principle of gas dynamic laser.
LICHTMAN and READY as well as GIORI et al. study the electron emission at laser radiation.
HONIG and WOOLSTON work with a mass spectrograph combined with focused ruby laser. These

high-performance experiments (1:10^3) are made on conductors (Cu, Mo, Ta, W, steel, graphite) and semi-conductors (Ge, Si); a non-conductor is also investigated.

MEYERAND and HAUGHT are the first to report on the air-discharge induced by the huge impulses of a ruby laser.

LEITH and UPATNIEKS use laser as a light source producing holography.

BAYLEY et al. deal with the measurement of the absorption ability of water (H_2O, HDO, D_2O) in the infrared range from 0.7 to 10 μm.

KAPANY, PEPPERS, ZWENG and FLOCKS perform animal experiments for the photocoagulation of the retina by ruby laser.

GOLDMAN et al. study the radiation effect of ruby laser on various tissues.

SAKS and ROTH – Microscopic studies on the effect of ruby laser radiation on the Spirogyra alga.

1964 PATEL observes laser oscillations in CO_2 gas. The wave-length of the strongest one is 10.6324μm. This first laser works with a constant voltage discharge tube of 5 m, filled with pure CO_2; the pressure is 0.2 torr. The continuous output is only 1 mW. By adding nitrogen (N_2) and helium (He) PATEL et al. manage to increase the output power significantly. Nowadays the CO_2 laser is one of the most efficient lasers.

BRIDGES describes the argon laser.

HARGROVE, FORK and POLLACK can establish the mode locking by means of a transductor built-in a helium-neon laser (acoustooptic modulation).

GEUSIC, MARCOS and VAN UITERT – Successful experiments with new combinations of host substances like rare earth metals. The yttrium-aluminium-garnet (YAG), $Y_3Al_5O_{12}$ is the best known among them.

CROCKER, GEBBIE, KIMMIT and MATHIAS explore the infrared for the laser.

RAMSDEN and SAVIC, RAIZER (1965) attempt to explain the air-discharge.

McGUFF et al. publish the first paper on the surgical application of the laser. They irradiate malignant human and animal tumours with laser impulses exclusively.

1965 MOELLER and RIDGEN realize that by adding helium to the mixture of the CO_2 and N_2 the efficiency increases.

WILSON (1966) obtains inversion in nitrogen stream through ultrasound-acceleration.

STAHLE and HOEGBERG – First application of the laser in otorhinolaryngology.

JAKO performs experiments with neodymium laser (constructed together with POLANY) on the vocal cords of corpses.

STELLAR (1965a, b) studies the effect of laser radiation on the brain and nervous system.

PEPPERS describes a ruby laser microscope designed for biological investigations.

HOYE and MINTON carry out the first bloodless liver resection of a rabbit by means of argon laser.

SOROKIN and LANKARD, when irradiating phtalocyanine solution with ruby laser, find out the laser-emitting ability of organic dyes. This is the first dye-laser.

DE MARIA, STETSER and HEYNAU use a reversibly decoloring agent in the resonator of the neodymium laser, thus ultra-short impulses can be induced (self-mode locking).

MICHON, ERNEST and AUFFERT perform mode-locking in a neodymium glass laser.

L'ESPERANCE, Jr. compares the photocoagulation produced by xenon arc-light and ruby laser.

YAHR and STRULLY perform experiments with CO_2 laser in dogs. This is the first surgical application of this type of laser.

1967 SOROKIN and LANKARD obtain excellent laser radiation in the visible spectral range.

WOOD and SCHWARZ – Passive quality locking in a CO_2 laser, with sulphur-hexafluoride (SF_6) absorber.

GIORDMAINE et al. develop the two-photonfluorescence (TPF)-technique for the measurement of pico-sec impulses.

SPENCER, LENZO and BALLMAN survey the dielectric materials for the electrooptics, elastooptics and ultrasound.

KOROBKIN et al. (1968) study the "spark" that occurs in the air due to focused laser radiation. GULLBERG, HARTMANN, KOCK and TENGROTH study the harmful effect of CO_2 laser on the cornea of rabbits.

1968 KOROBKIN and ALCOCK – Air-discharge experiments with ruby laser. Hypothesis of self-focusing.
HAGEN (1969) produces a 25 m-long line from air-discharge points with a high-radiance neodymium laser.
BASOV, KRIUKOV, ZAKHAROV, SENATSKY and TEHEKALIN observe neutron emission from lithium deuteride placed in the focus of ultrashort impulses of a high-power laser.
MAKOUS and GOULD publish an in-depth study on the effect of laser radiation of the human eye. The threshold of damage primarily depends on the heating effect.
L'ESPERANCE – The introduction of the argon ion laser into ophthalmology.
MULVANEY and BECK – The introduction of the argon laser into urology.
MULLINS, JENNINGS and MCCLUSKY report on a liver-resection by carbon dioxide (CO_2) laser.

1969 DUMACHIN and ROCCA-SERRA are the first to realize the principle of transversal stimulation in a CO_2 laser; the pressure of the gas mixture (CO_2, N_2 and He) can be increased to 450 torr.
TIFFANY, TARG and FOSTER construct a high-power gas transport CO_2 laser.
KUEHN and MONSON try to optimalize the parameters of a gas dynamic CO_2 laser.

1970 GOODAL et al. report on non-focused CO_2 laser irradiation for the control of bleeding due to gastric cancer and ulcer.
GONZALES et al. are the first to use the CO_2 laser in liver surgery.
MÜSSIGGANG and KATSAROS – Pioneering studies on the surgical application of neodymium laser.

1971 NATH develops a new light-conductor of great significance in the endoscopic use of laser. Continuous powers over 100 W and pulse-powers of megawatt range can be transmitted.

1972 NATH introduces this new light conductor at a surgical clinic in Munich and wants to develop it to a flexible laser-knife.
JAKO – Experiments on vocal cords of dogs; CO_2 laser combined with a ZEISS operation microscope is used. This is the start of the application of lasers in laryngeal surgery.
HALL, BEACH, BAKER and MORISON study by kinematography the cutting and vaporisation changes of tissues due to CO_2 laser irradiation.
BREWER: non-linear spectroscopy – Greater accuracy of the laser technique than ever before.
SHARON modifies the CO_2 laser as recommended by KAPLAN. The new instrument (SHARPLAN) is more convenient for surgical use.

1973 The first reports on the clinical application of the CO_2 laser: breast, plastic, and gynecologic (cervix) surgery.
BOYER reports on the preparations for provoking nuclear fusion by laser.
SLINEY and FREASIER investigate the ocular damages caused by modern light sources.
NATH, GORISCH and KIEFBACHER apply fibre-optics combined with argon or neodym-YAG-laser for endoscopy.
NATH et al. conduct argon laser radiation with flexible fibre-optics of a gastroscope.
GOLDMAN, NATH, SCHINDLER, FIDLER and ROCKWELL describe their experience with a high-power (max 200 W) neodym-YAG laser. The quartz fibre-optics developed by NATH and SCHINDLER, due to its flexibility and high transmittance (80%), proves to be a suitable transmission system. The objecting beam is provided by a helium-neon laser. A neodym-YAG laser is also investigated.
DREYFUS and HODGSON study in various gases the UV-laser stimulated by an electron beam.

1974 WALLACE and DREYFUS construct the first high-pressure xenon laser continuously operating in VUV range.
FRÜHMORGEN, REIDENBACH, BODEM, KADUK and DEMLING report on the effect of argon laser on the gastrointestinal tract.

GROTELÜSCHEN and BÖDECKER compare the suitability of CO_2 and neodym-YAG lasers as cutting devices.

MESTER et al. study the wound-healing effect of the laser.

1975 SEALER and HART describe the first inert gas halogenide laser; the stimulated emission of xenon bromide (XeBr) is at $\lambda = 281.8$ nm.

The first international symposium on laser surgery.

DWYER (USA) works with an argon laser ophthalmological coagulator combined with fibre-optics.

FRÜHMORGEN et al. in Erlangen-Nürnberg use commercially available argon laser equipped with flexible plastic light conductor.

KIEFHABER in Munich prefers the neodym-YAG to argon laser due to its higher power. Application in clinical endoscopy.

OHSHIRO (Japan) uses commercially available ruby laser modified by himself for treating patients with chromatic maculae.

The laser has a wide spectrum of application: non-linear laser spectroscopy, laser fusion, separation of isotopes, cell research (index of cellular migration, microirradiation, cell counting and classification), tumour destruction by photoactivation, ophthalmology, surgery, treatment of burns, otolaryngology, medical optic holography, cancer control, telecommunication for medical purposes, scanning and recording, data processing, computer systems, holocamera for meteorology.

1976 ASCHER and HEPPNER perform the first successful brain-tumour operation, with a Sharplan modified by them. They use helium-neon laser, and a zinc-selenium lense is substituted for a non-transparent germanium lense. The size of the microadapter is reduced. The surgeon controls the laser beam with a microscope-assisted sterile-covered switch-board (microslad).

VERSCHUEREN – Guiding publication on the CO_2 laser.

STAEHLER, HOFSTETTER and SIEPE initiate the cystoscopic treatment of bladder tumours with neodym-YAG laser at the University Clinic of Urology, Munich.

KOSLOW and MOSKALIK (Leningrad) report on 330 patients with early malignant and benign skin tumours, treated with neodym-glass laser.

1977 CASPERS – The application of helium-neon laser in acupuncture.

1980 In the frame of the NASA program natural laser irradiation was observed in the atomic sphere of the Mars.

1981–
1986 Rapid dissemination of the use of laser in the various fields of medicine.

Nobel Prize awarded for laser research:

1964 TOWNES, BASOW, PROKHOROW

1981 SHAWLOW, BLOEMBERGEN

2. The Physics of the Laser Beam

2.1. Introduction

Before giving a qualitative picture about the laser beam some basic data should be presented, without details of the quantum mechanics. The energy of the atom is determined by the electrons on the orbits. As to their state the electrons possess different energy levels with a definite quantity of energy per each. The transition from the higher E_a level to the lower E_b level results in an energy emission of $E_a - E_b$, in the form of light. According to PLANCK and EINSTEIN the light emission occurs at a specific frequency and a non-divisible quantity of energy called photon.

The frequency of the photon can be calculated by the Niels Borh's formula as follows:

$$T_{ab} = (E_a - E_b)\, h$$

$$T_{ab} = \text{photon frequency}$$

$$h = \text{Planck's constant} = 6.63 \times 10^{-34}\ \text{Js}$$

The wavelength λ_{ab}, $T_{ab} \times \lambda_{ab} = c$, $c = 3.000 \times 10^8$ m/sec the velocity of light. At collision the photons behave as elementary particles and are subject to the principle of the conservation of energy.

In the early part of this century, EINSTEIN described the conditions of light emission and the interaction between the light and the atom. He deduced three different interactions:

1. spontaneous light emission
2. light absorption
3. stimulated light emission.

2.2. Spontaneous light emission

The transition of nuclear energy from the E_2 to E_1 level takes place spontaneously. The photon frequency occurred can be expressed by the $(E_2 - E_1)\, h$ formula, as already referred to. The light, which results from spontaneous emission, scatters to all directions with equal probability. Its frequency is not ν_{21}, but spreads in a limited space having a ν_{21} centre as explained by quantum mechanics.

The light of an electric lamp occurs from spontaneous emission, the free excited electrons of the incandescent filament collide with the bound electrons, thus causing the transition of the excited atoms to a higher energy level. Then the spontaneous transition to a lower energy level results in a light emission (Fig. 1, 2).

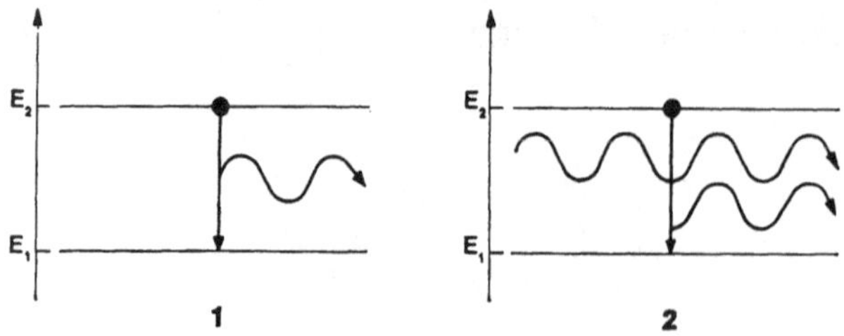

Fig. 1. The light emission

1. Spontaneous light emission
2. Stimulated light emission, $E_1 E_2$ = energy levels

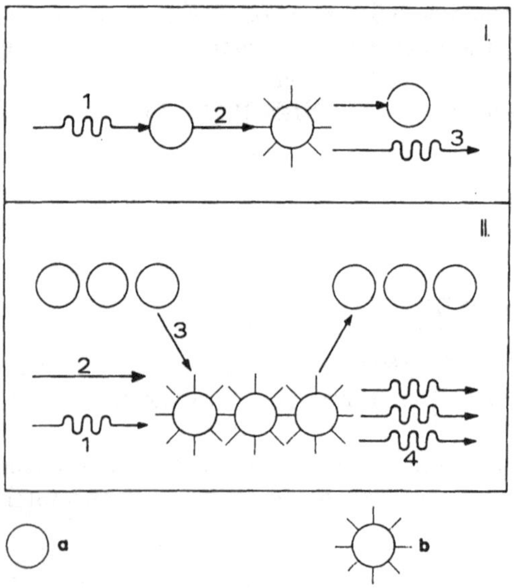

Fig. 2. Light emission and absorption

I. Spontaneous light emission, 1 = stimulation ray, 2 = absorption, 3 = spontaneous emission, a = equilibrium (E_1 level of energy), b = excitation (E_2 level of energy)
II. Stimulated light emission (laser), 1 = stimulation ray, 2 = energy excess, 3 = state of activation, 4 = laser beam, a = laser medium in equilibrium (E_1 level of energy), b = laser medium in excitation (E_2 level of energy)

2.3. Light absorption

Let us assume an atom at the E_1 low energy level, being collided with a photon of ν_{21} frequency. The atom absorbs the energy of the photon ($E_2 - E_1$) and the transition to the higher E_2 level becomes possible. The colourful sight of objects is explained by this phenomenon. When daylight falls on an object the latter absorbs one or two colours from the white light spectrum. The reflected light contains the complementary colours determining the colour of the given object (Fig. 2).

2.4. Stimulated light emission

There is a group of atoms of E_2 high energy level and of a very slow natural transition to the E_1 level. By stimulated emission this transition gives way to a ν_{21} photon, it collides with an excited atom, resulting in two ν_{21} photons of equal frequency. Both photons can stimulate another two atoms bringing about already four photons. The word LASER, *L*ight *A*mplification by Stimulated Emission of Radiation comes from this chain reaction. The light produced in this process is of the same frequency and direction as the stimulating light (Fig. 2).

2.5. Principle of the laser instrument

For easier understanding the principle of emerging of the laser beam we describe the operation of the ruby laser, the simplest type of laser instrument (Fig.3). Its laser medium is a synthetic ruby bar. Atoms of this ruby bar are activated by the flashes of the surrounding xenon lamp into transition to a higher energy level. This process is called optical amplification.

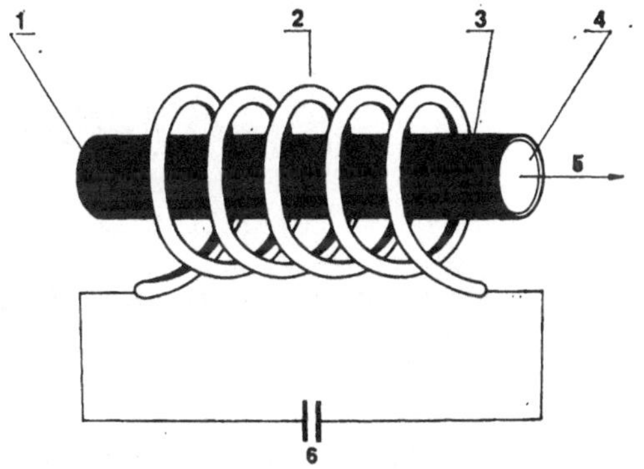

Fig. 3. Conceptual construction of the ruby laser

1. reflecting mirror, 2. xenon flashlight lamp, 3. laser tube (laser medium), 4. partially reflecting mirror, 5. laser beam, 6. source of energy

The majority of atoms being in stimulated state is called inversion mass. This laser is placed into an optical cylinder with mirrors at both ends. The two mirrors are coaxial. A few of the atoms of the inversion group emit photons into all directions at the spontaneous transition into a lower energy level. A part of the photons radiates along the axis of the cylinder, makes several passages, while being reflected to and from by the mirrors. These photons collide with the stimulated atoms in the ruby tube and stimulate them for emitting the same kind of photons into the same direction. Consequently, plenty of photons are emitted along the axis of the cylinder. This is the laser beam. Since one of the mirrors is semipermissive a part of the laser beams leaves the cylinder. The ruby lasers emit light impulses. Intermittently, the xenon lamp generates inversion atomic groups.

2.6. Properties of the laser beam

The individual laser beams are of the same wavelength. On the contrary, the wavelength of the white light as a mixture, varies between 0.4 and 0.8 mm. Lasers work in this range (Fig. 4). In spite of differences in the wavelength, energy and biological-biochemical effects, the various types of lasers have common physical properties. They are as follows:

1. Monochromatic and strongly bundled;
2. Slightly divergent (should be focused);
3. Enormous intensity (maximum: 500 MW/1 m^2);
4. Great coherence in time and space;
5. Highly polarized;
6. Generation of a very strong electromagnetic power;
7. Varying wavelength;
8. A part of the beam is absorbed while the other is reflected by biological tissues.

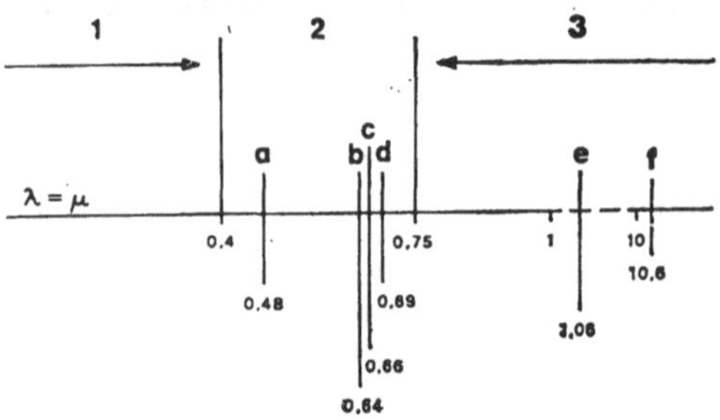

Fig. 4. Wavelength ranges of the light
1. ultraviolet, 2. visible, 3. infrared, a) argon, b) krypton, c) helium-neon, d) ruby, e) neodym-YAG, f) CO_2

The physical properties of the laser light are primarily distinguished from those of the common one by its coherence, monochromatism and high density of power.

Coherence (Figs. 5 and 6)

- Coherence in time
  Due to the stimulated emission in the cavity, the photons leaving the cavity are all in phase.

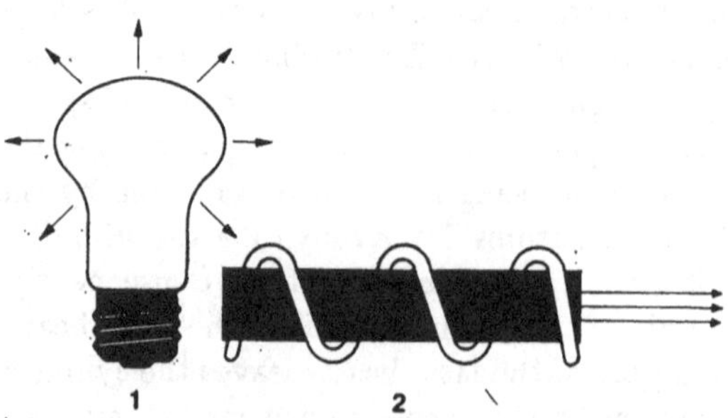

Fig. 5. 1. incoherent source of light, 2. coherent source of light

- Coherence in space
  Due to the mechanism in the cavity, the laser beam is also spatially coherent, i.e., at any time the phases are equal across a wavefront.
  Leaving the cavity, the laser beam is a narrow and parallel bundle.

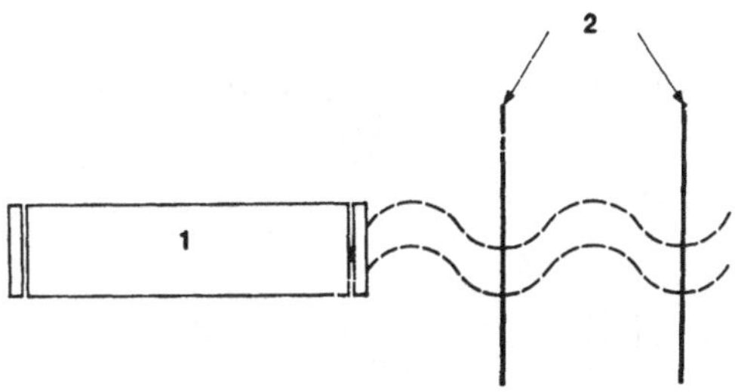

Fig. 6. The spatial coherence
1. laser, 2. wavefront planes

Energy density and power density

The cross section of the parallel beam leaving the cavity has a certain surface. The energy density is the total amount of energy passing per unit surface of the cross section, and is expressed in joule/cm². The energy density is a convenient denomination as far as pulsed lasers are concerned, since the very short duration of their pulses (about 1 millisecond) does not compel us to take the time factor into consideration. Contrarily when speaking about continuous wave lasers (devices delivering an uninterrupted beam) it is better to use the power density (often called intensity), which is expressed in joule/cm² × second or watt/cm².

Due to their high degree of coherence, laser beams can be focused onto a very small spot with an energy density considerably higher than in the parallel beam. The importance of the coherence can be illustrated by comparing an electrical 100 W bulb with a CO_2 laser producing 100 W. Trying to focus the white light from the bulb with lenses, will only yield a fraction of the emitted light energy at the focus, since the bulb is emitting light in all directions. Conversely the whole coherent beam from the CO_2 laser can be focused onto a spot thus generating enough energy to burn a hole in an asbestos brick.

2.7. The structure and type of laser instruments

Each laser instrument consists of three parts: (Fig. 3)

- active or amplifying medium (laser substance)
- source of energy
- optical resonator (optical cavity) or feedback system (see Fig. 7)

As to the amplifying medium four types of lasers are usually distinguished:

a) Solid lasers in which the active substance is an evenly distributed "contamination" in a solid matrix. E.g., in a ruby laser the laser medium consists of chromium ions embedded in a bar-shaped alumina crystal.

b) In gas lasers a gas (e.g. argon) or a mixture of gases (e.g. helium and neon) are filled in the discharge tube.

c) Liquid lasers contain a solution of an organic or inorganic dye, e.g. alcoholic solution of eosin.

d) Semiconductor lasers usually operate with crystal diodes, e.g. gallium arsenide.

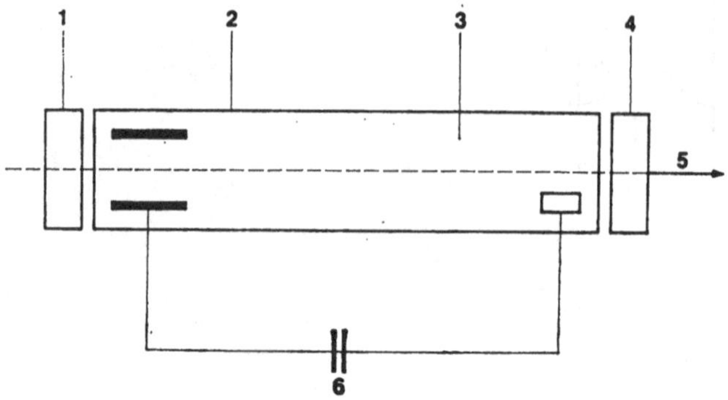

Fig. 7. Laser oscillator
1. totally reflecting mirror, 2. optical resonator, 3. **active medium**, 4. partially reflecting mirror, 5. permitted ray (laser beam), 6. source of energy

The functional prerequisite of a laser instrument is a sufficient amount of stimulated atoms (or ions or molecules) of the active medium, that is, population inversion should be established. This means that the overwhelming majority of atoms is in a stimulated state compared to normal conditions when most of the atoms are non-stimulated, i.e. a reversed distribution exists at the two levels of energy.

The laser medium is stimulated by an outer source of energy which is, in most instances, a common flash lamp of high power.

The gas lasers are supplied with electric current. The amplification of light is solved by feedback through an optical resonator which consists of two mirrors. The laser beam is reflected by the mirrors thus passing through the active medium several times and is amplified by induced emission. The amplified bundle of light leaves the system through the semipermissive mirror.

The lasers can be run in continuous or impulse operation. The ruby laser emits at a wavelength of 694.3 nm. The duration of a single flash is about 0.5–1 ms in the simplest pulse operation and the radiation energy of a flash is 1–30 J.

The helium-neon (He-Ne) gas laser radiates in red and infrared, its strongest spectral line is at 632.8 nm. The He-Ne lasers operating continuously provide 5–50 mW power depending on their size. Due to its great coherence the laser light can easily be focused, therefore concentrated on a surface of a diameter of about 0.0005 mm. This renders possible the application of the high-energy lasers (CO_2, Neodym-YAG) as surgical knife.

3. The Biological Effects of Lasers

3.1. Specific laser effects

The effect of the high-energy laser is independent of the properties of the material irradiated. It is because the highly concentrated energy instantly evaporates almost everything on the surface of the given object. This heat effect is non-specific and is exclusively the function of the density of power at the target. The huge order of concentration of energy available by laser is, however, of extremely short duration.

There is a difference between the biological effect of impulse and continuous operation lasers: the intervals between impulses enable some reparative processes, to act on the contrary, this is impossible during continuous operation.

One of the most important parameters of the biological effect is the absorption coefficient of the living tissue which depends on the wavelength of the laser beam. The absorption and reflection change conversely. It is well known that atoms, molecules, etc., absorb definite frequencies in the whole range of the spectrum selectively.

Since the living tissue is optically heterogeneous certain components of the tissue are especially sensitive to monochromatic radiation. According to their colour the tissues absorb at different spectral wavelengths and in case of equal powers the greater biological effect can be expected of the frequency coinciding with that of the absorption range of the tissue. Eventually, the selectivity of biological effects is determined by these relations. The biological effect is therefore considerably influenced by the blood supply of the individual tissues, i.e., the grade of ferrous or other sort of pigmentation.

There might be an analogy between the mechanisms of the biological effect of the laser and the ionizing radiation. It has been detected that these two types of radiation can cause an additive effect. Doses of laser and ionizing radiation, separately, without any biological effect, were lethal to cell cultures when applied simultaneously (ROUNDS et al. 1979).

a) The retinal epithelium of rabbits, the pigmentous and non-pigmentous versions of melanoma and fibroblastoid elements of mice were compared. It was observed that cells were damaged or destroyed by laser effect, depending on their pigment content. Non-pigmented cells could be destroyed only after vitally staining them, e.g. with Janus-green which sensitized them towards ruby laser irradiation.

b) The contractility of the heart, smooth and striated muscles decreases due to laser irradiation, indicating the inactivation of ATPase by photodynamic effect.

c) As a result of laser treatment endothelial cells of rabbits grow into multinuclear giant cells. In addition, the chromosome analysis shows fragments and dicentric shapes. This refers to the damage of the mitotic apparatus. Since this change is maintained in subcultures as well it bears evidence for the mutagenicity of the laser.

The tissue culture is the most suitable object for studying cell organs and chromosomal changes. It can be completed by sensitization with vital staining which considerably increases the absorption of the ray.

The light microscope is necessary for distinguishing the living and dead cells while the phase-contrast microscope is more convenient for detecting the alterations of the cellular structures. Temporal cellular changes can be most suitably followed by microkinematography. The morphological changes can be studied by electron microscope which provides much better resolution than the former ones. The biological effects are recently investigated by biochemistry, autoradiography and cytochemistry as well. Their findings concerning the cellular functions and structure can be summarized as follows:

a) In multicellular plants a part of the plasmodesma of the mitella axialis was removed by a ruby laser microbeam of 156 μm diameter, then microdrops of oil were injected to the cytoplasm. After several expositions the cell grew more rapidly than after a single treatment but did not reach the growth rate of an untreated cell (Saaks and Roth 1963).

b) The irradiation of monocellular systems and cells of higher organisms can be used for studying intracellular communication and "cellular oecology".

c) Rabbit embryoblastomers of 8- and 16-cellular stage were treated with ruby microwave, following vital staining. Detachment of certain blastomers could be produced in vitro. Maternal chromosomes could be separated from similarly treated fertilized frog-spawn, then the embryos developed a haploid syndrome.

d) The effect of ruby-, neodymium- and argon lasers was most extensively studied on various cell organs in tissue cultures, among others on mitochrondria, RNA-synthesis and cytoplasm of fibroblasts and heart-muscle cells. Selective lesions as well as alterations in enzyme functions occurred due to the combined effect of radiation energy and vital staining.

e) In order to study the irradiation effect on the nervous system some authors irradiated the supra-oesophageal ganglion of spiders by a ruby laser beam of 7 μm diameter. The treatment resulted in a disturbance of the cobweb formation. Stimulation was obtained by argon laser treatment in the abdominal ganglion of the sea-Aplysia californica.
Mester et al. (1970) revealed that ruby laser irradiation could increase the production of acetylcholine in the Auerbach's plexus of the ileum of guinea-pigs. This method seems to be feasible to gain knowledge of cellular interconnections.

f) McGuff et al. (1964) performed oncological experiments with ruby laser.
   - Various human adenocarcinomas were transplanted into the cheek pouch of hamsters and 2 to 3 weeks later half of the animals were treated with a ruby laser impulse of 100 J energy as well as with He-Ne continuous irradiation in mW order of magnitude, for several hours. The tumours treated disappeared in an average of 27 days.
   - Malignant melanoma was transplanted into hamsters. In 17 controls the tumour persisted for 8.5 months, while the 18 treated animals became tumour-free in

about 20 days. The amelanotic and melanotic melanomas respond in the same way.

The experiments show that the selectivity of a laser beam depends on the wavelength, pigmentation, translucence, the blood supply of the tumour as well as on the ratio of the size of tumour and the dose irradiated.

- Hoye et al. (1966), when irradiating tumour transplants with neodymium laser of high energy, observed living tumour cells in the resultant steam. They reimplanted these cells into other animals. Thus, tumorous cells which are not completely destroyed can get into the neighbouring tissues and disseminate due to the high pressure.
- Rounds et al. (1979) succeeded in producing synergistic effect both in vitro and in a clinical case with the combination of ruby laser and X-irradiation. Cytostatic drugs, e.g. cyclophosphamide can increase the effect of laser, and thus with this combination, lower energy not inducing dissemination to the adjacent tissues serves for the destruction of the tumour. These experiments provide favourable information for selecting appropriate wavelength, power density and other combinations in the clinical practice.
- Mester et al. (1970) studied the effect of ruby laser in vitro on the growth of Ehrlich ascitic tumours. The growth rate, mitotic index and electron microscopic picture of animals were compared to controls inoculated with non-irradiated cells of the same donor. Following inoculation of the irradiated cells a shorter survival was observed than in the control group.

g) The effect of ruby laser on the bacterium phagocytosis of leukocytes (*Staph. pyog. aureus*) was under investigation. It was established that a radiation energy of 0.05 J/cm^2 considerably increased the bacterium phagocytosis of the white blood cells while a dose of 4.0 J/cm^2 markedly inhibited it.

h) The solutions of methylene blue and Janus green enhance the radiosensitivity of white blood cells while acridine orange alleviates it. The serial low doses applied to native WBC affect as an inhibitory high energy. This effect is mostly regarded as a ferment effect.

i) The potentiating effect of low energy irradiation and inhibitory effect of the high ones were witnessed in the hair growth of $C_{57}B$ and white mice, too. The weekly irradiation of 1 J/cm^2 applied for 3 to 5 weeks increased the hair growth while 10–11 irradiations caused inhibition. Also in this case a cumulative inhibitory effect was observed with the low doses.

The biological effects of fractionated irradiations summed up even if temporally prolonged. After a longer treatment inflammatory, then atrophic histological changes developed on the hair follicles. Following 15 treatments certain parts of the epithelium became wider due to the basal cell proliferation. This might already be regarded as a preblastomatous phenomenon, but after 30 irradiations it developed into atrophy, in consequence of the summation of effects. During this time some alterations became manifest in the visceral organs of certain animals, e.g. subcapsular coagulative cell necroses involving several layers in the liver. In three mice necrosis in the wall of the small intestine close to the anterior abdominal wall and secondary peritonitis occurred. It is understood from other experiments that the liver and the intestines are sensitive to direct high energy laser irradiation. Laser irradiation significantly accelerated the healing of a complete skin defect of 10 mm diameter artificially produced on the back of white mice. It is likely that the laser beam exerts a stimulating effect on the cellular activity at the edges and the base of the wound, increases the number of cell divisions and accelerates the production of the granulation tissue. It was observed by microscopy that the number of the dividing cells was greater in the treated area and the wound cavity filled up more speedily.

j) In view of the fact that the intestinal mucosa is very sensitive to radiations the effect of laser on its micromotility and the movement of intestinal villi – in situ – was taken under examination. It has been observed that the lower energy (1 to 3 J/cm^2) increased the automative movement of the intestinal villi while the higher energy inhibited, moreover stopped it. The application of about 7 J/cm^2 energy already shows some signs of destruction. It is supposed that in the automation-increasing effect of radiation the ganglia play an intermediary role.

k) Concerning the biological effect of the laser it was long ago suggested that, in addition to the heating effect, it might be attributed also to the ionizing radiation energy. To approach this problem two test objects especially sensitive to radiation were selected:

- Experiments upon dogs showed a transitional increase in the micromotility of intestinal mucosa for a low-dose (2 J/cm^2) laser energy. This effect is suspended or strongly reduced by the previous parenteral application of aminoethylthiouronium (AET).
- The stimulating or inhibitory effect of the laser beam is decreased by AET also at the bacterium phagocytosis of leukocytes. This protects the SH radical of thiol ferments against the damaging ionizing radiation effect.

These findings, therefore, support the explanation as to the mechanism of action of laser might be, to some extent, similar to that of the ionizing radiation.

Although plenty of data have been accumulated their interpretation is extremely difficult and numerous investigations are still needed for the definitive clarification of the results. It is indisputable, however, that the biological effect of laser far exceeds the opportunities offered by the ultraviolet and ionizing microbeams known as yet. There are further *potential fields of its application.*

The laser emission spectroscopy is based on the fact that from e.g., the biological material under investigation a cellular component becomes vaporized due to the intensive heat effect of the focused beam. The stimulated emission spectrum of this vapour can be fixed on a photosensitive film. This method is in-between the common optical spectrochemistry – which is suitable for the imaging of substances of 5 mm in width – and the X-ray microprobe the resolution of which is 1 μm.

a) The diameter of the laser beam is generally 50 μm and it is also suitable for the analysis of the intracellular cations of tissues (e.g. Ca, Mg, Cu, etc.).

b) The flow microphotometry is based on the application of a scattered laser beam.

The coherent beam of the He-Ne laser can be well used for measuring the bacterial proliferation. Some authors followed e.g. the colony formation of *E. coli* for 4 hours.

c) This technique was further developed, thus it has become suitable for determining the size of mammalian cells in a flowing suspension. This technique was applied for measuring the DNA content of cell populations, protein content of cells in tissue cultures and for detecting viruses in infected cells by immunofluorescence. Normal and tumorous cells could be recognized in a tumorous tissue by measuring quantitative differences of the DNA content. The effect of irradiation could also be detected in X-irradiated cells.

d) Biological application of holography. A three-dimensional picture of an object can be made by holography by dividing the bundle of a laser beam into two parts. One part called "object beam" reflects from the object onto a photosensitive plate while the other called "reference beam" reflects from a mirror onto the same plate, without touching the object. Interference occurs between the two beams and its picture is fixed on the photosensitive plate. This picture is influenced both by the phase- and amplitude parameters of the beam modulated by the object. In order to obtain a three-dimensional picture the object has to be illuminated by the coherent and monochromatic laser light of the same wavelength. Thus, viewing from a special direction a real and a virtual reconstructed picture can be seen. Especially in ophthalmology, this highly encouraging technique has the following main fields of application:

- Storage of three-dimensional pictures;
- Detection and three-dimensional presentation of pathological changes, e.g. retinal ablation, intraocular foreign bodies, etc.;
- Storage of information. One hologram can store the structure of the whole eye by a single exposition, and – if needed – can present the individual layers or the possible changes of contours. The movement of the eardrum can experimentally be studied by He-Ne gas laser because this technique is suitable for detecting even 10^{-10} to 10^{-5} cm of oscillation.

3.2. The aspecific effects of laser

When the laser beam of high energy (CO_2, Neodym-YAG) absorbs in the tissues it heats the irradiated area to several hundred degrees (C°). Since the heating that accompanies absorption occurs very rapidly and the heat conductivity of the neighbouring tissues is very small, the heat effect is localized to the area of irradiation. Due to the high temperature the tissues immediately get vaporized, meanwhile at the edge of the cut a necrotic zone is formed in the direction of the decreasing heat effect. At the hit point of the laser beam – at several hundred degrees – the structure of the target tissue is significantly modified. At 100°C the cellular fluid is boiled, and at several hundred °C several chemical reactions occur (denaturation of proteins, carbonization, combustion, etc.). The composition of the gas formed during these reactions varies with the tissues. During operations the gaseous endproducts have to be removed by a vacuum system for two reasons:

1. Good visibility of the operation area has to be provided.
2. Contamination of the operating theatre has to be decreased.

At the edge of a laser wound several zones can be microscopically distinguished. These are as follows (PLENK et al., 1979):

1. zone of carbonization
2. zone of coagulation necrosis
3. transitional (demarcation) zone
4. zone of hyperemia and oedema.

The depth and the relative size of these zones depend on the structure of the treated tissues and on the properties of the laser applied.

Living tissues absorb beams of the CO_2 laser much better than those of the Neodym-YAG. Due to this difference the CO_2 laser makes a sharper wound surface though the power applied is smaller – more than 20 watts – and the zone of the thermal damage is less deep. The Neodym-YAG laser can be used for cutting over 130 W, and it has a definite hemostatic effect as well. The zone of thermal damage can be decreased in both cases by applying an increasing frequency of the laser beam between 0.3300 and 10,000 Hz instead of irradiation with a stable frequency. Properties of the wound surface also depend on the duration of exposition and the width of the bundle of beam.

The cutting depth of the laser beam can be calculated according to the Goldman-Rockwell equation:

$$x = \frac{(1 - R) \times P \times T}{F \times p \times (L + c)} \text{(cm)},$$

where

x = cutting depth

$R(l)$ = reflectivity of the tissue

$P(w)$ = energy applied

$T(s)$ = time of exposition

$F(\text{cm}^2)$ = wound surface

$p/g\ (\text{cm}^2)$ = depth of the transection

$L(J/\text{g})$ = vaporization heat of the tissue

$c\ (\text{J/g °C})$ = specific tissue heat

(°C) = difference between the temperature of vaporization and that of the body.

In practice, however, it is sufficient to consider only the type and power of the laser, the type of the tissue, width of the cut and tension of the tissues. Our knowledge is not comprehensive enough about the response of tissues to laser irradiation therefore we are going to deal only with that supported by experimental data. The controversial findings will also be referred to.

3.3. System 400 CO_2 Surgical Laser used in our clinic

The System 400 CO_2 Surgical Laser operates at the infrared (invisible) wavelength of 10.6 microns. Laser power is continuously adjustable to 25 watts at the tissue site. The CO_2 laser beam functions parallel with the operator's line of sight when viewed through an operating microscope. A helium-neon (HeNe) laser with a red beam is coincident with the CO_2 laser beam and provides a visual aiming dot at the treatment site. This HeNe aiming beam is permanently aligned with the invisible CO_2 beam (Fig. 8).

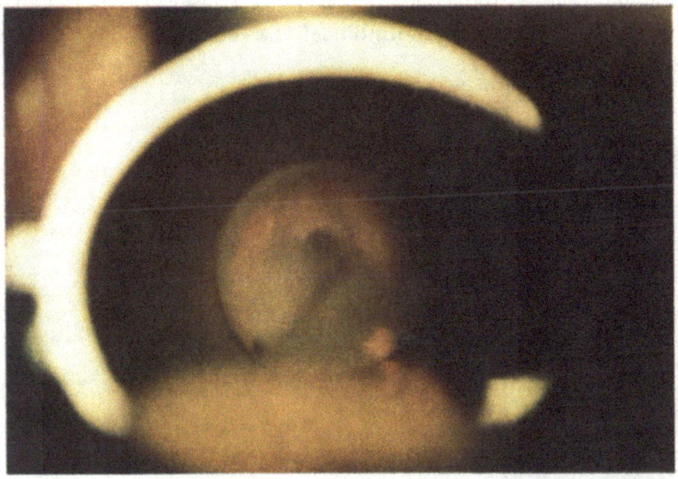

Fig. 8. The red He-Ne pilot light (endolaryngeal exploration)

The CO_2 laser light is focused at 400 mm (in focus with the microscopce objective) through its own optical system and delivers a treatment spot 2 mm in diameter. Optional lenses are available to provide 300-mm (spot size 1.5 mm) and 200-mm (spot size 1 mm) focal lengths. The degree and depth of tissue destruction is controlled by the amount of laser power delivered and the exposure time – both controlled by the physician. Exposures of 0.1, 0.2, 0.5, 1.0 second and "continuous" are available on the System 400. Exposure is initiated by a foot switch.

The CO_2 laser tube is a double-wall glass tube with integral laser mirrors. The double-wall construction allows water to circulate for cooling of the tube. A mixture of carbon dioxide, nitrogen and helium gas is fed to the tube from a gas bottle and evacuated from the tube by a vacuum pump. The high voltage for the tube is supplied through the umbilical from the control console along with gas and water. An electrical discharge in the tube much like that in fluorescent light excites the CO_2 gas molecules so that they will give off photons of light energy which are in the infrared part of the spectrum. These photons of light energy are amplified by the mirrors at either end of the laser tube, providing the output energy for therapeutic use. The small helium-neon laser tube and its power supply are housed in the laser head. An optical system is used to combine the helium-neon beam with the CO_2 beam so that the two are coaxial. An electronically controlled shutter deflects the laser beam into a power meter whenever this shutter is in the closed position. When the foot switch is depressed, the shutter flips out of position allowing the laser beam to go along the optical path to the target tissue for treatment.

A small vane attached to the shutter interrupts a photocell and light arrangement so that position of the shutter can be monitored by the safety circuits in the instrument. Should the shutter jam, either open or closed, the system will detect this and indicate a shutter malfunction on the front panel while turning off the laser at the same time.

Tissue destruction results from the rapid absorption of the infrared laser beam into the intra- and extra-cellular water in the tissue. Only the tissue at the focal point of the CO_2 laser beam is vaporized, leaving adjacent tissue virtually unaffected.

Instrument description

The System 400 Surgical Laser (Fig. 9) comprises the laser head, which attaches directly to a standard Zeiss operating microscope, and a control console. The laser head is attached to the control console by a single, multi-purpose umbilical that contains power cables, coolant conduits and gas lines (Fig. 10).

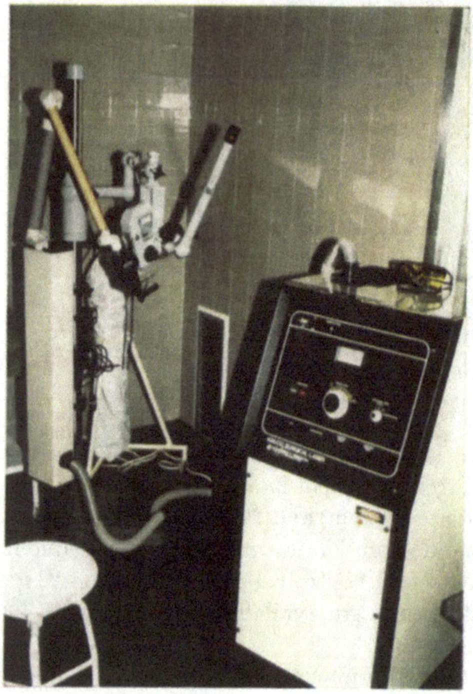

Fig. 9. The system of Coherent 400 CO_2 surgical laser

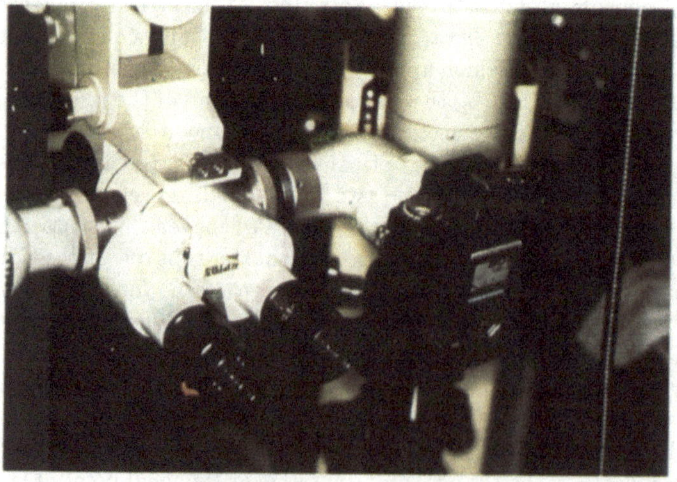

Fig. 10. The Zeiss OPMI-1 operating microscope

a) **Control Console:** The console contains the electronics, the self-contained cooling system, and the controls to turn the laser on and off and to set laser power and exposure settings. A storage well is provided on top of the control console for the laser head. Casters on the console allow it to be easily moved to the operating site (Fig. 11).

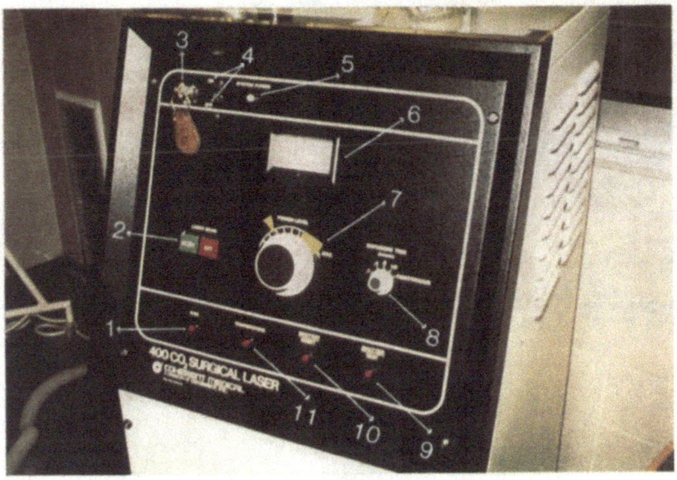

Fig. 11. Control console of the System 400
1. Low gas pressure indicator light, 2. Laser beam Ready/Off switches, 3. Master key switch, 4. System power On/Off switch, 5. System power indicator light, 6. Power level meter, 7. Power level control, 8. Exposure time control, 9. Test switch, 10. Shutter reset switch/light, 11. Coolant temperature indicator light

b) **Laser head:** contains the helium-neon laser and the CO_2 laser. Both beams are parfocal with the microscope, permanently aligned, and need no adjustment. Also contained in the laser head is a shutter that controls CO_2 laser exposure. The HeNe laser light (red) shows constantly when the LASER BEAM READY button is illuminated. A micromanipulator moves a mirror permitting precise positioning of the laser at the operating site. A manual safety shutter is located on the laser head adjacent to the microscope. This must be open (down) to permit the laser beam to reach the operating site. The manual safety shutter may be closed to block the beam and avoid unintentional exposure.

c) **Counterbalance:** There are two counterbalances to facilitate adjustment of the microscope. One counterbalance fits over the top of the microscope stand elevator column and serves to offset the additional weight of the laser head. The other counterbalance supports the laser head and assists in movement and focusing of the microscope.

d) **Foot switch:** Stepping on the foot switch (Fig. 12) activates the laser. The duration of the laser exposure is determined by the time preset on the EXPOSURE TIME control. Releasing the foot switch will interrupt the exposure. With the EXPOSURE TIME control on "continuous", the foot switch alone controls exposure time.

e) **Two-stage gas regulator:** This regulator is supplied with the system. The primary gauge shows the gas pressure in the cylinder, ~2 000 psi (13 790 kPa) when new. A valve adjusts the secondary pressure to the proper system operating pressure of 20 psi (140 kPa).

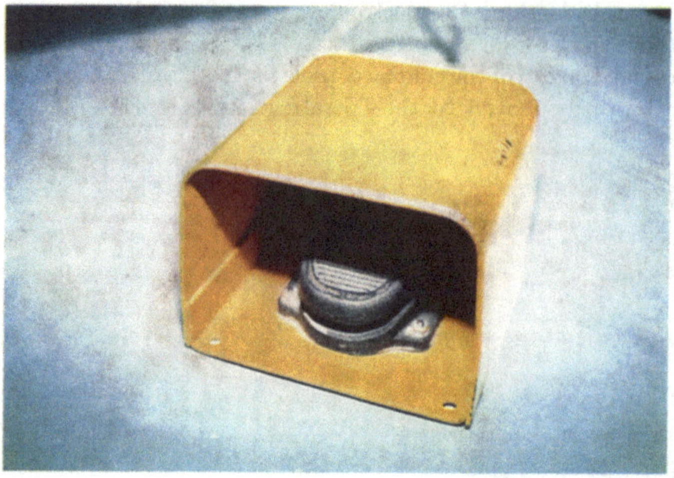

Fig. 12. Foot pedal

Specifications

Laser Power: Continuously adjustable to 25 watts at tissue site
Laser Wavelength (CO_2): 10.6 micron, infrared-invisible
Focal Length (and spot size): 400 mm (2 mm) standard; 300 mm (1.5 mm) and 200 mm (1 mm) optional
Exposure Time: 0.1, 0.2, 0.5, 1.0 second and "continuous"
Power Requirements: 117/220 volts AC, 50/60 Hz, 15/7.5 amps
Cooling: Closed cycle, water-to-air heat exchanger, self-contained in control console
Coolant: Distilled water and 3 drops Algaetrine algaecide. Capacity: Approx. 5 pints (2.37 litres)
Gas Mixture: Premixed carbon dioxide (4.5%), nitrogen (13.5%), and helium (82%)
Gas Cylinder: Replaceable cylinders, available commercially, size 3 or 30 A, 30 cu. ft. (0.85 m^3) with CGA 580 valve
Aiming Device: Visible red helium-neon laser beam (0.8 mw, 632.8 nm)
Micromanipulator: Ambidextrous, 25-mm-diam. sweep (Zeiss), or 20-mm sweep (Leisegang)
Shipping Weight: 395 pounds (179.19 kilograms)

f) **Gas Cylinder:** A Number 3 or 3O A cylinder/30 cu ft. or 0.85 m^3 will fit inside the control console and is recommended for use. A commercially available laser gas mixture of 82.0% helium, 13.5% nitrogen, and 4.5% carbon dioxide is used as the lasing medium. The valve must be a CGA-580. Cylinder colour code is brown, yellow, white. Cylinder pressure at 70°F (22°C) when full, should be 2000 psi (13790 kPa). In normal usage, a cylinder should last from six months to a year.

g) **Laser Head Mounting Plate:** The plate and screws necessary to mount the laser head to the microscope are included with the laser.

h) **Microscope** (Fig. 10): Only the Zeiss OPMI-1S, and OPMI-6 operating microscopes are recommended for use with the System 400. The Zeiss microscope must be fitted with a 400-mm focal length objective lens, since the laser beam itself is focused at this point (unless the Accessory Lens Kit is ordered for focal lengths of 200 and 300 mm).

System Controls and Indicators

CONTROL OR INDICATOR	Function
MASTER KEY SWITCH	Prevents unauthorized use of the laser.
ON/OFF SWITCH	Circuit breaker which turns system power on and off when MASTER key switch is ON.
SYSTEM POWER INDICATOR	Light goes on to indicate power to the system. (Does not indicate on/off status of the laser beam.)
POWER LEVEL METER	Calibrated to read power delivered to the treatment site when the shutter is opened. Deactivated during exposure.
POWER LEVEL CONTROL	Adjusts power at tissue site from 0 to 25 watts or greater.
EXPOSURE TIME CONTROL	Selects exposure times of 0.1, 0.2, 0.5, or 1.0 seconds, or continuous exposure.
COOLANT TEMPERATURE INDICATOR LIGHT	Indicates when the coolant flow is inadequate.
SHUTTER TEST SWITCH	Used to test shutter and timing circuits.
SHUTTER RESET SWITCH/ LIGHT	Indicates a system fault. Press to reset and reactivate system.
GAS PRESSURE INDICATOR LIGHT	Indicates low gas pressure. (System will not operate.)
LASER BEAM READY/OFF SWITCHES	Press READY to turn on CO_2 laser, the HeNe laser, and ON light found on laser head. Press OFF to turn off same.

Controls on Laser Head Only

MICROMANIPULATOR	Used to position laser beam on operating site.
MANUAL SAFETY SHUTTER	When it is down, it is open; when it is up, it is closed.
EMISSION INDICATOR LIGHT	Indicates laser emission is possible when this light is on. Avoid eye or skin exposure to direct or scattered CO_2 laser light.

Operating Instructions (Including Daily Checkout Procedure)

a) Check the coolant reservoir to make sure that coolant level is adequate (filled to the line indicated).

b) Turn on gas cylinder valve at least 1/2 turn counterclockwise and verify adequate gas for your procedure. The CO_2 cylinder can be left on all day, but should be closed clockwise after the day's last procedure. When open, the primary pressure gauge should read in the range from over 2000 down to 200. If the pressure is less than 200 psi (1379 kPa), erratic operation may result. Change gas cyliners.

c) Place key in master ON/OFF switch and turn to ON position (Fig. 11). This key is removable only in the OFF position for safety; the laser is not operable when the key is removed.

d) Turn the system ON with the ON/OFF switch to the right of the key switch. This brings power to the entire system and lights the SYSTEM POWER indicator on the control console.
e) If the red SHUTTER RESET button is on, press it.
f) Press green LASER BEAM READY switch. (LASER READY light should come on.)
g) Adjust the gas regulator until the secondary pressure reads 20 psi (140 kPa). The unit must be in LASER BEAM READY mode for this.
h) Set EXPOSURE TIME to desired setting.
i) Set POWER LEVEL to desired power after observing the POWER LEVEL meter.
j) Open the manual safety shutter on the laser head by moving it to the down position.
k) Adjust microscope in accordance with manufacturer's instructions.
l) Make any adjustments that may be required for EXPOSURE TIME and POWER LEVEL.
m) Use micromanipulator to direct the laser beam to the treatment site.
n) Step on foot switch to activate laser. Releasing the foot switch will interrupt the exposure if the full preselected time is not desired. When the EXPOSURE TIME control is set at "continuous", the foot switch alone controls exposure time.
o) Turn laser beam OFF if procedure is interrupted. System power may be left ON. To resume treatment, turn laser beam on (READY).
p) Turn SYSTEM POWER OFF after each complete procedure. If it is the last procedure of the day, close valve on gas cylinder, then release all tension on the pressure-adjusting handle in the centre of the regulator by turning it counterclockwise until it turns freely.
q) Turn master key switch OFF and remove key to prevent unauthorized use.

Checkout Procedure

a) With the laser in the READY mode, set exposure time to 0.1 second.
b) Point the aiming beam (the red HeNe laser) at a safe medium such as wet gauze or cinder block. Step on the foot switch and observe that the CO_2 laser is operating.
c) To test safety circuits, set exposure time to any preset interval, but NOT to "continuous".
d) Press TEST button and hold it down.
e) Depress the foot switch and hold until exposure is completed.
f) The system should go into a "fault mode", in which the following things will happen:

TURNED OFF	TURNED ON
CO_2 laser	LASER BEAM OFF indicator
Helium-Neon laser	SHUTTER RESET lamp
Vacuum valve	
ON lamp located on laser head	
LASER BEAM READY indicator	

g) If a fault is NOT produced, check to make sure "continuous" was not set as the exposure time. If it was, reset as in c) above, then repeat steps d) and e).

h) If the fault has been accomplished without problem, reactivate the system by pressing the SHUTTER RESET button and the LASER BEAM READY button, in that order. Proceed with operating step h).

3.4. Laser and the microscope

In the technical, biological and medical application of the laser the microscope has various **advantages**:

a) the object and the processes induced by the laser are well observable;
b) precise positioning of the laser;
c) the laser effect can be induced on a very small spot;
d) The laser action can be monitored by a TV-set, in addition to the microscope.

There are two sorts of combinations of the laser and the microscope:

a) The laser and microscope are closely united: laser microscope, microlaser system, etc.
b) The laser is adopted to an ordinary microscope by an accessory instrument: microscope adapter.

In each case a safety interblock should protect the surgeon's eyes from the laser radiation.

Concerning the optics high technical requirements must be met. For the protection of the lense the flow of an inert gas is frequently applied.

The operation microscope combined with laser (Fig. 10)

The operation microscope (OPMI) is very helpful to the physician, makes his work possible and easier. It has been successfully applied in ophthalmology, otolaryngology, neurosurgery and gynaecology for a long time.

Since simultaneous or common observation and documentation are required, numerous attachment units, tubes, photoadapters are needed for monitoring the moving processes. Some auxiliary instruments adjusted to a black-and-white or colour TV set permit a larger audience to follow the operation. A few of these units are joined or connected to a distributor. In the case of photo- or film-adapters an automatic shutter control is useful; it is appropriately set according to the intensity of the reflected light.

The optics of the operation microscope is constructed in a way that preferably a great distance can be left between the operating site and the objective, thus ensuring enough space for the operating physician. This is to be maintained during the operation as well. Regularly, the space for work has to be equal with the focal distance of the objective applied.

The working field can be illuminated coaxially with the microscope or slantwise; the mono- or dual slanting illumination is recommended when strongly reflected or poor-structured surfaces are concerned. An incandescent or halogen lamp can be used as a source of light and mounted on a tripod to keep the microscope far enough from the developing heat. The intensive light is directed on the operative site by total reflection through a flexible fiberoptics. This cold illumination system is also space-saving because no lamp container is needed adjacent to the microscope.

The blow-up V of an operation microscope depends on various factors. When the focus of an objective is f_{obj} and the focus of the tube is f_{tub}, γ is the medium blowing factor of the blowing switch (for rapid blow-changing during operation) and the own blowing effect of the ocular called V_{oc}, the following equation is valid:

$$V = \frac{f_{tub}}{f_{obj}} \gamma V_{oc}.$$

The f_{tub} is 125 or 160 mm for Zeiss microscopes. There are 5 grades of the Galilei-switch that can be handled manually, the scale units by γ values 6, 10, 25 and 40 are 0.4, 0.63, 1.6 and 2.5. The "lane" refers to position 16, then γ equals to 1. The Zoom-system exists either on the manual or the electric part and can be controlled without switching in the range of $0.5 \leq \gamma \leq 2.5$ – that means a blow-change of 1:5 at the Zoom-system.

When applying the laser combined with operation microscope special auxiliary units are needed:

a) **Adapter for the microscope**
It establishes a direct contact between the operation microscope and the laser. The laser can be attached to the adapter by means of an articulated arm. The parallel beams conducted to the adapter box will be focused at the entry, by means of an exchangeable lens, then reflected to a small movable mirror. This reflects from above, i.e. the incident radiation directs to the target area.

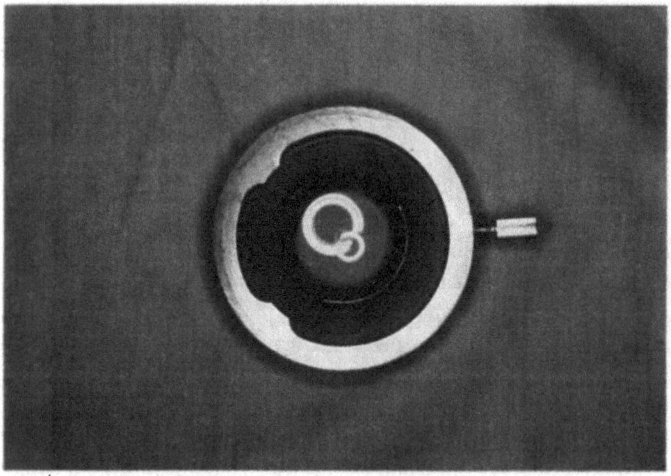

Fig. 13. Adapter to a camera

b) **Target-indicating laser**
The area that is to be affected by invisible infrared radiation must be made appreciable by means of a visible light. For this purpose the red light of a small power He-Ne laser or the bluish-green light of the argon laser is used. The pilot-light emiteted from these auxiliary sources is conducted in the same way as described for the working rays of the CO_2 laser (Fig. 8).

c) **Control-console** for the surgeon
In order that the operating physician can set and change the direction of radiation when looking into the operation microscope, he should drive a micromanipulator or a joystick by hand or electric current. When the pilot light is well visible and set

for the target, the surgeon activates the laser by the foot switch and the laser "shoots" It is highly advantageous to locate all the supplementary units on an aseptically coverable control-console ("microslad").

3.4.1. Handpiece

The laser instrument can be used not only with a microscope but as a handpiece as well (Fig. 14).

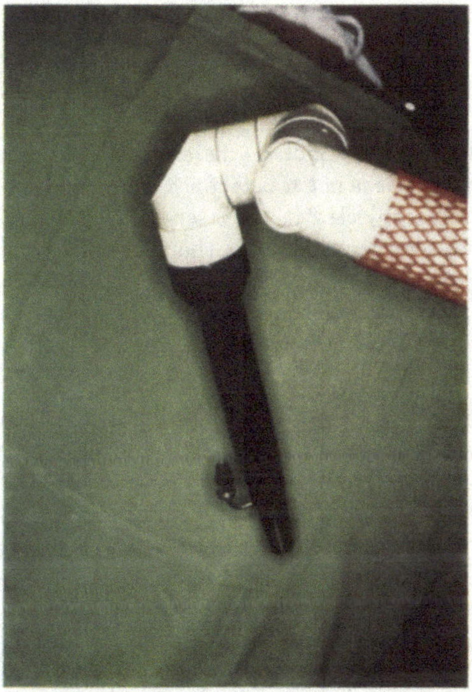

Fig. 14. Handpiece of the 400 CO_2 surgical laser

After the detachment of the microscope a handpiece can be adjusted through an adapter. The properties of the CO_2 laser beam coming through the handpiece are equal with those described above. The handpiece is movable in space by an articulated system and approaches the operating site to about 2 cm. The handpiece is sterilizable in gas. The invisible beam of the CO_2 laser is made visible by He-Ne red laser.

3.5. The advantages of the surgical application of the laser

The ideal wound-surface would be that having a minimal zone of heat damage with a maximal hemostatic effect. From this point of view, the present, most commonly used lasers (CO_2, YAG, Argon) are superior to the electrocauter. (Considering the recent technical research trend even more favourable sources of laser are expectable to be used in medicine).

a) At the moment of cutting – depending on the power – the **vascular walls** in the necrotic zone of the wound surface become obstructed through **coagulation** (GROTELÜSCHEN and BUCHHOLZ, 1978). This refers to the diffuse, hemophilic bleedings. It generates two important benefits of the laser:
   - In case of vessels with a diameter of less than 2 mm a bloodless wound surface can be operated on, which is a great advantage from operation technical point of view, when hypervascularized organs (liver, brain, kidney, etc.) are concerned.
   - The obstruction of the lymphatic vessels seems to be an even more considerable advantage. It can decrease the metastasis formation which may be provoked in the radical tumour surgery even when taking the principle of "no touch operation" in view.

To prove the above, various research groups performed model experiments. The majority of them conformed the significant decrease in the tumour cell dissemination (FRISHMAN et al., 1974 and PELED et al., 1976).

Certain observations, however, suggest an inhibited tumorous dissemination also in case of such narrow necrotic zone when the hemostasis is not satisfactory. There are controversial results, namely in case a dye solution is injected in the laser-induced wound 48 hours following surgery the dye granules can soon be detected in the macrophages of the regional lymph nodes. PLENK et al. (1979) and EHRENBERGER and INNITZER (1978) suggest that, under certain circumstances, the blood vessels are sealed by the laser while the lymphatic ones are not. To gain a more precise knowledge of this process further investigations have to be undertaken.

b) The coagulation of the blood vessels prevents the spreading of bacteria, too. Depending on the focusing of the different laser beams when cutting with the laser scalpel the instrument does not touch the operative field, and no tumour tissue or bacteria adhere to it. In addition, the laser beam heats the wound surface to several hundred °C, consequently the wound remains sterile (STELLAR et al., 1974).

   In the surgery of infected areas and under warlike circumstances this technical property may have definite advantages since the wound is sterile and the instrument needs no sterilizing. The no-touch application means an atraumatic surgical technique as well.

c) The laser incision does not cause edema and the scar formation is minimal.

d) Several investigators establish that the laser procedure reduces the postoperative pain (KAPLAN 1976, CHRISTENSEN 1976).

e) The operation microscope ensures an exquisitely precise targeting and an absolute hit safety (to µm order of magnitude).

f) Further significant advantages are the preservation of normal tissue structures, the performance of function-preserving operations and the very simple surgical procedure.

3.6. The disadvantages of the surgical application of the laser

These disadvantages are of technical and economic character. The handpiece of the laser ("laser scalpel") is attached to the laser instrument through a spatially movable articulated system. It weighs through brakes on the operating hand, which means a burden, the joints are sluggishly movable. Therefore it can be used in the deeplying tissues with difficulties. Further inconvenience and visual disturbance are caused by the suction tube hanging onto the operative field, which ensures the suction of gases and body fluids. The dryness of the wound surface is important because the fluid on its top better absorbs the laser energy, thus instead of the linear evaporation of the wound surface tissues the whole wound surface gets heated. The laser operating team must observe the safety regulations regarding their own and the patient's clothing, the movements in the operating room as well as the isolation of the operative field and the laser instrument.

The eyes of the patient and the operating team as well as other parts of their body must be protected with spectacles and clothing, respectively. It especially relates to those instruments where the laser beam is not focused and can transmit its whole energy to any material getting in its way. In case of focused beams the area beyond the focal point is less endangered. In order to avoid undesired injuries the operative field at the line of incision must be protected from the stray beam. These rules must be kept since the laser injuries are relatively frequent. FRIED (1984) inquired about this 229 laryngo-surgeons using the laser, and evaluated the answers of 210 filled-in questionnaires. According to 153, surgical laser was used averagely 6 times a month. Hundred and three surgeons did not observe accessory injuries, 49 witnessed complications (one of them performed 700 operations). The highest number of complications was 15. Their occurrence increased with the number of interventions. Altogether 81 postoperative complications were mentioned. The most frequent ones were the often fatal endotracheal explosion (28), burns on the face (9), pneumothorax (5), bleedings (3), subcutaneous emphysema (2). Although the majority of the surgeons asked were elderly and had a great professional skill the apparent simplicity of the laser technique sometimes lulled their attention. Then the loose handling of the rules led to certain complications.

The technical difficulties of the surgical use of the laser were reduced by more recent instruments.

In view of the intensity of laser research the elimination of the technical disadvantages can be expected. Besides all the above the high costs of the laser instrument and the need for highly qualified professionals are also disadvantages. Therefore the application of the laser is justified only in institutions selected specially for this task.

3.7. The indications of the surgical application of the laser

Since the advantages of the laser are of therapeutic, the negligible disadvantages of technical and pecuniary characters, its application is particularly desirable and indicated in certain fields of surgery. These are as follows:

1. Surgery of angiomas
2. Surgery of malignant tumours
3. Surgery of organs with abundant blood supply (liver, kidney, tongue, etc.)
4. Operations performed in case of altered blood coagulation (hemophilia, thrombocytopenia, anticoagulant treatment)
5. In case of infected operative field, decubitus
6. Endoscopic microsurgery
7. Cardiac, brain surgery
8. Surgery of patients with pacemaker.

4. Clinical Application of the Laser

The common feature of the primary head and neck tumours is that their regional metastases develop in one of the cervical lymph node chains. Since the surgical treatment of the tumorous process is successful only by the simultaneous removal of the primary and its cervical metastases, furthermore, the primary tumours extend far beyond the boundaries of the individual specialities of medicine, the developed countries established the head and neck surgery. This new branch of surgery is on the margin of otorhinolaryngology, the general, oral and plastic surgeries. It deals with the complex treatment (operations, radio- and chemotherapy and their combinations) of all precanceroses, benign and malignant tumours situated between the clavicle and the base of the skull.

Considering that the use of the surgical laser is principally indicated for oncological reasons, in this section of our book the classical ORL region is extended and the head and neck laser surgery is also dealt with.

The head and neck surgery is already a classical field of the laser surgery, too. The primaries here are visible (skin, lip, tongue, bucca), they are easily explorable (nasal cavity, mesopharynx, larynx) or they are situated relatively superficially (parotis, thyroid gland). The highly disadvantageous adaptation difficulty of the laser is almost negligible here, thus the handpiece and the microtechnique are easily applicable. Beyond that the advantages of the laser are excellently enforceable.

4.1. The surgery of skin tumours

The dermatooncosurgical use of the laser is hard to be discussed separately from the dermatologic or plastic surgical application, especially when the incision of the skin lesion is concerned. The skin defect can be treated in various manners, depending on its size and type. In case surgical procedures are used for the esthetic and functional reconstructions, it is called plastic surgery. When applying the laser technique the laser is used for vaporization or excision while the defect is reconstructed by plastic surgical methods. Considering that the skin of the head and neck regions is especially important from the esthetic point of view the plastic surgical results should be the best attainable after the laser removal of the tumours. Aronoff (1976) regarded those patients as suitable for laser operations who had hematopoietic organ diseases, who had overcome prior chemotherapy or turned to a physician due to any lesion ebulking on the body surface. Later, this modest circle of indications got wider. Cutaneous lesions of practically any size or histological type can be removed by laser and the skin defect reconstructed by one of the numerous plastic surgical methods available.

It was first published by Hoye and Minton (1965) that the high energy, continuous laser beam could reduce the bleeding on the cut surface. Subsequently, Mullins et al. (1968) and Fiadler et al. (1975) conducted a great number of experiments on the bloodful parenchymatous organs (liver, spleen) and the skin of smaller and bigger animals (e.g. dogs). Statistically it became evident that from the hemostatic point of view the laser causing the least damage on the cut surface is superior to the electric knife.

Experimental results

4.1.1. The characteristics of the laser operations on the skin

According to comparative clinical studies the feature of the wounds inflicted by the CO_2 laser, the Bovie knife or the scalpel significantly differs. The scalpel e.g. iduces about 4-fold blood loss than the CO_2 laser. From this point of view the CO_2 laser is also more advantageous than the Bovie knife. The blood loss ratio of the laser, electric knife, scalpel is 1:1.7:3.3. Levine et al. (1975) claim that an operation with the CO_2 laser is 1:1.37 faster than that with an electric knife but 1:0.67 slower than with a scalpel. Others describe the ratio of the duration of surgery with scalpel/electric knife/laser = 1/1.2/1.6. The power of the laser used was 1–5 kW/cm^2 and 5–20 kW/cm^2. These authors believe that the longer duration of the laser surgery was due to technical causes. Similarly, the duration of operations also differs with argon and Neodym-YAG. For the excision of 10–20% of the adult total body surface (TBS) about 2,000–4,000 ml of blood substitution is necessary. The volume of blood required and the duration of the operation vary with the parts of the body, i.e. in case of thoracic or abdominal wounds of 18% TBS considerably less blood should be replaced than for limb wounds of the same TBS. In case of equivalent percent of TBS an adult loses more blood than a child. The operative loss of blood and body fluid also depends on the condition of the patient's hematopoietic system, the extent of the edema developments and the secondary infection occurred as well as on the duraton of the operation. Since the absorption coefficient of the CO_2 laser for tissues is excellent the loss of fluid and blood can be diminished. The operative field should be kept dry because the tissue fluids and blood on the wound surface also absorb the laser beam, thus its heat effect on the tissues weakens. The lateral traction of the cut surfaces is advantageous in case of the laser operations since prior to the transection the smaller blood vessels get tight, their coagulation is better (there is less blood in a narrow lumen), the incision is quicker, the direction of intrusion is more precise and the deep-lying structures are easier to recognize. With increasing the energy (over 60 Watt) the heat effect of the beam on the surrounding tissues decreases, and consequently, so does the coagulation of the vessels. With a lower power (20–40 Watt) the wound surface is dryer and the laser scalpel is more effectual. Investigations have proved that the incidence of wound superinfections is the highest when using the scalpel, then the laser beam and electric knife follow. Depending on the condition of the skin the lasered surface comprise, in addition to the smoke-steam generating with the evaporation of extra- and intracellular fluids, various organic and inorganic substances, bacteria and fungi, too. The latter may get into the laser smoke also from the area not evaporated yet. (The elimination of the infectious materials must be solved for the protection of the patient and the staff of the operating theatre – special isolation, operation clothing, exhaustor.)

4.1.2. The duration and quality of wound-healing

The clinicians should be absolutely familiar with the wound healing following the laser incision or excision. The wound cut by the laser can be sealed in two different ways: with sutures or autografts. A smaller laser-made wound can be sealed primarily. It is feasible to use atraumatic, monophilic suturing materials, to drain the wound cavity and to control it frequently. Several authors have found that the healing of laser-made wounds is though of good quality but prolonged in time. Experiments on the back of rats have shown that wounds made by electric knife took 40 days to reach the tearing strength of a scalpel-made wound. In case of a defect of 2 cm^2 the contraction and epithelization of the wound were 20% lower with electric knife after 2 weeks and the wound healing was only 95% even after 28 days (HISHIMOTO et al. 1975). FIDLERS's (1974) experiments on scalpel-cut wounds suggest that neither the epithelization nor the survival of the skin transplant seemed more favourable than with the lasing. Larger defects can definitely be closed with skin grafts from other parts of the body. The autograft covers the defect, protects it from being superinfected, decreases the further loss of the liquid components of blood as well as decreases the patient's heat loss.

Instead of autografts allografts can also be used. When using a mashgraft the allograft is stretched to 1.5, 2, 3, 4, 6-fold of its original size, then soaked and placed into the defect. It is advisible to avoid using suturing materials, devitalized tissues, etc. since they prevent the development of the microcirculation. The most successful solution is provided by the mashgraft on the esthetically (face, neck) or functionally most tender parts of the body. Following the laser operation the dressing and further management of the wound covered with a skin graft do not differ from the traditional procedure. The same refers to the pre- and postoperative treatment of the patient.

Histological examinations have been performed to study the incorporation of the autograft. Following the use of an electric knife a huge amount of blood components have been found on the wound surface. On day 4 following surgery a fibrinotic plate full of erythrocytes and fibrinoblasts as well as inflammation of the adjacent tissues could be observed between the cut surface and the autograft. With a laser incision the wound surface was almost entirely bloodless and by day 4 the fibrinoblastful wound surface and the autograft stuck closely together. The plate between them and the inflammation of the environment could not be detected. By day 8 the healing of the skin was perfect, while only partial when using electric knife. Since the wound healing seems a bit prolonged, after the primary wound sealing and transplantation the sutures are recommended to be removed some days later than usual.

4.1.3. Clinical application

4.1.3.1. Benign tumours and skin lesions. Angiomas

The hemangiomas and lymphangiomas situated on different parts of the body are problematic from the point of view of extirpation, the CO_2 laser is well suitable for their treatment. At the moment of cutting it closes the blood vessels to 1 mm diameter while to 2 mm – after preliminary strangulation – coagulates them. The larger vessels at the line of intersection are also easier to recognize and to manage. Therefore excisions have been made with CO_2 laser on various vascularized tumours like e.g. on purulent granulomas, acquired angiomas, on angiomas occurred in blue vesicular naevus syndrome, superficial varicositis, facial teleangiectasias, lymphangiomas and in case of Rendu-Osler-Weber hemorrhagic teleangiectasias.

In patients with blue vesicular naevus syndrome the tumour often regressed after surgery with scalpel and high frequency electric knife.

Regression and continuous healing of angiomas have been observed with the use of various laser types (pulsing ruby, neodymium and CO_2 lasers). After extensive CO_2 laser incisions and primary wound closure the majority of tumours regressed. The wound of a CO_2 laser extirpation of angiomas on the face (including the eyelid), the palm and heel recovered with excellent cosmetic results. Japanese plastic surgeons removed large volume growing cavernous agniomas including Kasabach-Merrit syndromes on the skin of children, with minimal bleeding. In case of similar operations, after removal of the extensive vascular tumours, the disturbances of cardio-vascular functions caused greater problems than the bleedings.

For the treatment of port-wine spots the argon laser is more suitable than the CO_2 one. No satisfactory cosmetic result was obtained with the CO_2 laser – in the treatment of web-like teleangiectasia on the thigh or of the superficial varicosity not even if an operation microscope was attached to the CO_2 laser. This instrument ensures small and clean-cut medical points. Rather frequently, deep white straight scar developed. Despite this the CO_2 laser has recently been tried on similar teleangiectasias of the face and nose, and favourable results have been achieved. The same experience could be seen with surgical laser in lymphangiomas. For a male patient with relapsing extended lymphangioma after 4 conventional scalpel operations the CO_2 laser could bring about recovery. Within the next 24 months the tumour did not recur.

After removal of several tumours the healing of the wound took place with scarring, the healing was sometimes incomplete, the hemangioma persisted or relapsed. The same operation with argon laser gave better results. For this reason, some surgeons (e.g. ARONOFF, 1981) evaporated the larger part of the tumours with the CO_2 laser, then at the edge of the defect they used argon laser for completing the operation. Thus the wound healing was scar-free, the incorporation of the allograft was unperturbed, the plastic results improved.

4.1.3.2. Verruca vulgaris and condyloma acuminatum

In the recent years CO_2 laser has been used at the laser laboratory of the Cincinnati Medical University for the treatment of the verruca vulgaris and condyloma acuminatum also including its giant form of Buschke-Lewenstein. Beside the liquid nitrogen, cryotherapy, podophyllin, Euphorbia and other cytostatics, the CO_2 laser also has been used as adjuvant therapy in the treatment programs of warts. Verruca was removed in 45 patients via vaporization with an operation microscope-assisted CO_2 laser. The patient group comprised those with persistent and recurrent as well as immunosuppressed extensive warts. The CO_2 laser was not used as first-choice treatment but after other methods had proved unsuccessful. During an observation period of 6 to 36 months a 75% remission was observed in 45 treated patients. On the perlingual area a residual scar remained after the removal of the warts with CO_2 laser. The CO_2 laser instrument attached with operation microscope is advantageous for treating warts because the verrucous tissue can be easily separated from the healthy one.

When treating 10 patients with condyloma acuminatum with CO_2 laser no recurrence was observed for 10 to 34 months. Scarring was minimal or none. To evaluate the CO_2

laser removal of the condyloma acumination high frequency electrocoagulation was used as control on the same lesion. One side was lased while the other coagulated. Not only smaller bleeding but better cosmetic result were provided by the CO_2 laser.

4.1.3.3. Cutaneous malignancies

4.1.3.3.1. Epithelial tumours

The majority of epithelial malignancies are situated on the head and neck region. The most frequent histologic type is the non-metastasizing basalioma, considerably rarer are the metastasizing keratinizing or non-keratinizing squamous cell carcinomas or other histologic types encountered. Their treatment is principally the radical surgery, sometimes cryotherapy, radiotherapy or their combination. The greatest advantage of the radical surgery performed with laser is that the beam closes the lymphatic vessels at the moment of cutting, thus the danger of the tumorous spread in case of metastasizing histologic types is decreased. In addition to this – due to the special esthetic situation of the head and neck region – the quality of wound healing and the graft-accepting ability of the wound are also noteworthy.

In case of a small tumour not involving the deep-lying structures the laser removal of the cutaneous head and neck malignancies is technically extremely simple. The only, though general oncosurgical problem is to define the distance of incision from the macroscopically intact edge of the tumour (Fig. 15a, b, c).

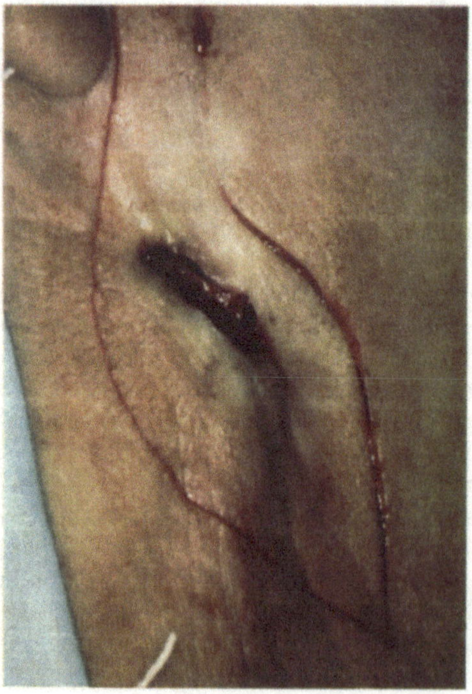

Fig. 15a. Extended basal cell carcinoma of the neck

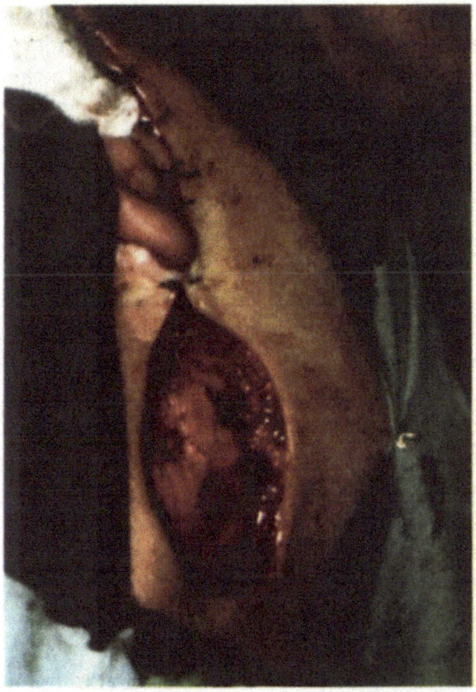

Fig. 15b. Condition after laser excision (partial wound closure)

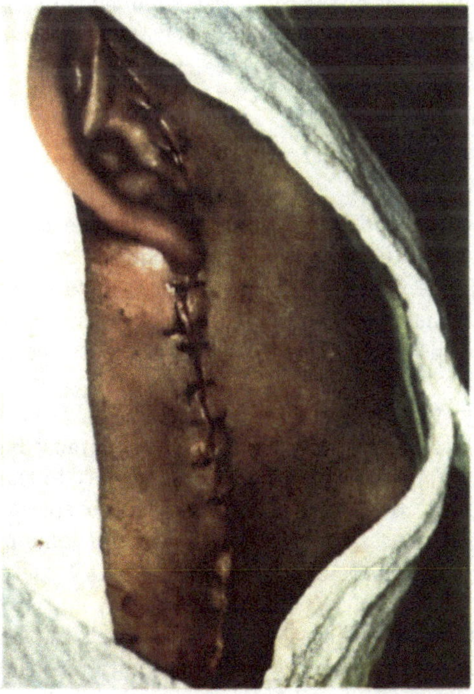

Fig. 15c. Condition after complete wound closure

The first cutaneous tumours removed by CO_2 laser were the basal cell carcinomas, especially those occurring with profuse bleeding on the sunburnt skin as secondary poikilodermas. Comparative incisions with scalpel and laser were made to evaluate the volume of bleeding and the healing on these hypervascular, atrophic, teleangiectasis skins. Although the bleeding was inconsiderable, the wound healed slower. On the sunburnt skin the wound mark was cosmetically not as satisfactory as with the application of cold knife. When using the CO_2 laser as a cauter excellent scars were obtained.

The basal cell carcinoma removed with laser recurs much later than in case of other methods. The initial experiences indicate that the incidence of late metastases of epithelial cancers slightly diminishes following laser operations. The deepness of involution does not mean an unsolvable task. The extirpation only depends on how deeply one can reach the underlying structures with the handpiece. The large, deforming defects caused must be closed in these cases, too. The reconstructive plastic surgical procedure differs from the conventional one only as to the laser defect of the cut surface. The radical laser surgery of deep-involving cutaneous head and neck tumours is demonstrated on a few patients treated by ARONOFF (1976). The widely extended epithelial cancer on the scalp and face of a female patient with poor general condition has been persistent for 10 years, despite the surgical and irradiation treatment. The tumour on the skin was removed with surgical laser, the frontal bone, the orbit and the dura were resected. The scalp was mobilized onto the site of the defect. The Silastic prosthesis placed around the dural injury ensured good contour. The suture lines healed perfectly but an inflammation developed on the adjacent part of the prosthesis, which through a meningitis, led to the patient's death. The multiple cutaneous cancer of a patient with chronic lymphoid leukemia was treated with cryotherapy. On the cryodestructed region a generalizing inflammation developed. Thereafter the patient had to be resuscitated. Subsequently, one part of the tumour involving most of the scalp was removed conventionally, the other part with laser, and the defect was closed. The laser operation was impressive, the bleeding minimal and the wound healing agreeable, respectively.

4.1.3.3.2. Malignant melanoma

The malignant melanoma originating from any melanin-containing organ of the body is perhaps the most malignant histologic type. It is extremely dangerous since it metastasizes not only in lymphatic but also in hematogenic ways and thus develops metastases early to various lymph nodes and distant organs, too. There is no successful mode of therapy available for this disease as yet. The success of therapy is doubtful, the death rate of patients is extremely high.

As a rule, its first-line therapy is surgery, then radio- and chemotherapy or their combination may be applied. When operating the primary tumour the incision must be made on the edges far (3 to 6 cm) from the tumour in the normal tissues, deeply to the fascia. The principle of no-touch isolation must be followed, which means a special technical difficulty. Otherwise the intraoperative massaging and pulling of the tumour may result in the detachment and lymphogenic-hematogenic spreading of the loosely connecting tumour cells.

When considering that the laser can close the lymphatic and blood vessels at the moment of cutting, and is applicable in a no-touch way from afar – in addition to the advantages mentioned previously it seems to be an ideal tool for the removal of melanomas.

The main lines and movements of the excision of melanomas are identical with the surgery of squamous cell carcinomas.

It is a difference, however, that the incision must be made farer from the tumour and the edges of the wound are to be moved carefully by hooks. If no radical operation is possible it is feasible to use the laser for vaporization.

The quality and duration of the wound healing, the mode of wound management do not differ from the other cutaneous laser operations. The area of primary and regional lymphatics are irradiated postoperatively with 60 Gy, and cytostatic agents (e.g. DTIC) are administered. If regional metastases occur regional node dissection (RND), while in case of generalization total body grid irradiation (TBGI) may be performed.

The success of the oncological application of the laser is still disputable. The number of cases is low, the follow-up period is short, therefore there is a wide range of opinions. Some clinicians accept the application of the laser as favourable, others – though not denying its advantages – have not experienced oncological benefit. Our own limited number of operations is neither suitable for definitive evaluation.

4.2. Auricular tumours

The laser operations of auricular tumours are indicated in similar cases as described in the chapter of cutaneous malignancies. In addition, the chondromas are also suitable for laser surgery. The laser operations of the auricle are technically extremely difficult and dangerous because in case of superficial lesions the cartilages must be saved. Since the laser beam is not suitable for anatomical preparation it is advisible on the area con-

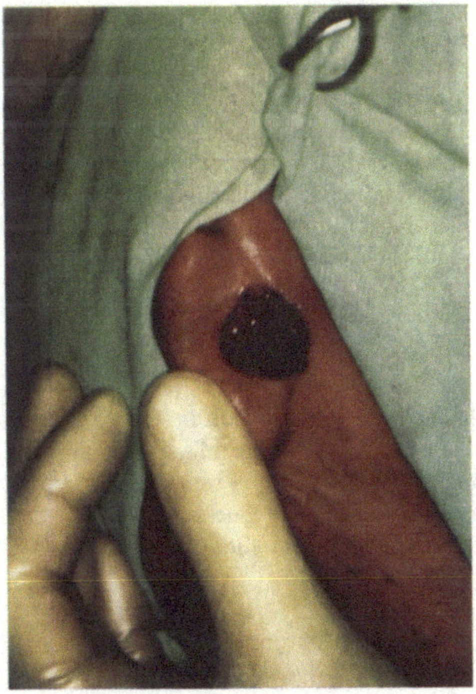

Fig. 16a. Basal cell carcinoma of the auricle

cerned, to conventionally separate the perichondrium from the skin and the mucosa, to perform its preparation, then in perichondrial protection to carry out the laser excision or vaporization. This procedure is followed by the plastic reconstruction (Fig. 16a, b).

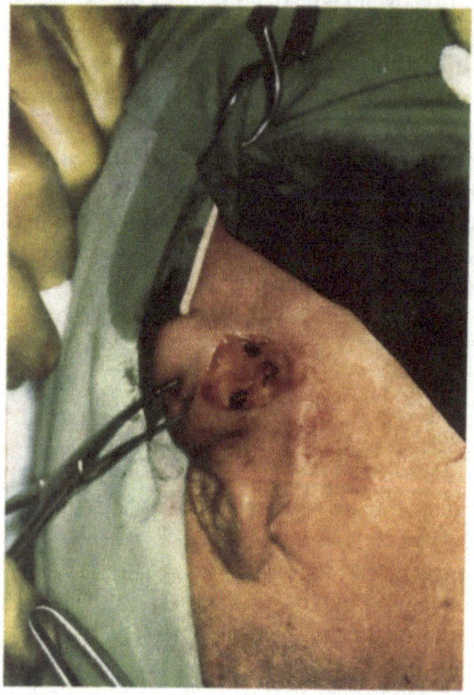

Fig. 16b. Condition after laser excision

When the tumours infiltrate the cartilages of all the three layers, the oncological considerations are of principal importance. The cartilage is resected together with the skin, then the skin of the incision line is separated from the cartilage and, prior to the reconstruction, the heat-destructed chondric edge in about 2 mm distance is cut with a cold instrument. In case of isolated chondromas the skin must be separated first from the tumour with conventional instruments, and then comes the laser incision.

4.3. Nasal operations with laser

The laser has manifold excellent properties that make its application in the rhinologic surgery most attractive. Among them the hemostatic ability, the absence of damage to the surrounding tissues, the minimal postoperative edema, rapid wound healing with minimal scar tissue formation are noteworthy. In view of these favourable characteristics the use of laser is getting more and more widespread in nasal surgery.

4.3.1. External laser operations

Due to general operative technical causes (see chapters on the advantages and indications of the laser) the extranasal laser operations with handpiece are indicated in case of the epithelial-pigmentous and vascular tumours of the nasal skin and different histological types of the chondrous frame.

In the extranasal interventions all considerations detailed in the chapter of cutaneous tumours are valid. Furthermore, the protection of the nasal cartilage or, in case of infiltrating primary tumours, its resection are essential points. Perichondrial operations are technically similar to the auricular ones. The importance of avoiding the heat damage to the cartilage and the secondary sterile necrosis is especially emphasized in rhinophymas.

The rhinophyma is the condition of progressive nasal increase resulted from the hypertrophy of soft tissues especially of the sebaceous gland. Its precise cause is unknown as yet. Different surgical techniques are described, including the tissue excision with total skin transplantation, elevation of the skin and subcutaneous tissue excision, subtotal excision with scalpel or blade, which is followed by reepithelization from the remaining epithelial glands. One common drawback of the methods enumerated is the abuse bleeding hindering the good visibility, the precise excision and the performance of a smooth transition on the surrounding skin.

These problems can mostly be overcome by the use of operation microscope and CO_2 laser suitable for microsurgical excisions. The hemostatic effect of the laser and the excellent wound healing are great advantages to the treatment of rhinophymas.

The cutaneous surface is washed with hexachlorophenic solution, then dried. The eyes are covered with saline-moistened pads and, except for the other parts of the face, the nose is covered with multilayer wet gauze.

The metal instruments are kept far from the operative field, to prevent the reflection of the laser light. The further safety measurements are identical with those described earlier.

One per cent lidocaine with 1:100,000 epinephrine is injected in the nasal skin. The laser is set for manual control and pedal start. The laser power can be set in the range 10 to 50 W.

The bigger mass of the tissue is cut with the laser. The increasing quality of the remaining tissue is evaporated under microscope until the necessary depth is reached. This depth is indicated by the quantity of sebum that can be pressed out of its dilated duct. The assistant periodically presses the nostrils and expresses the sebum from the gland. When it comes hard, the necessary depth is attained. The gradual removal of the edges of wound ensures a smooth transition to the normal tissue. Care must be taken to leaving a continuous skin ledge around the nostrils, to avoid the contradiction of the necessary scar.

The hemostasis is excellent, without remarkable bleeding.

The nose is inuncted with bacitracin ointment. There is no need for prophylactic or therapeutic antibiotic treatments.

The postoperative complaints are minimal. Within 24 to 48 hours dark burn slough develops but vanishes in 10 days. The complete epithelization takes place in about 3 to 4 weeks. The follow-up experience of many authors shows superior cosmetic results to those after conventional operations.

The laser handpiece can be applied with success also for the extirpation of far-advanced, disseminated tumours as well. Outstanding therapeutic result was seen also in a patient whose upper lip, lower wall of the maxilla, septum and one wing of the nose were removed with laser, then the defect was reconstructed with cutaneous flap. The course of disease of a 86-year old female patient is also instructive. She was admitted to hospital in poor performance status with pulmonary edema and fibrillation and recurrent nasal tumour infiltrating the orbit. The base of the orbit and its lateral wall were removed with laser. Although the operation was most probably of palliative character, the original complaints of the patient (constant bleeding and flow) could be ceased. In another patient radical neck dissection and radical extirpation of the primary tumour were performed with surgical laser due to carcinoma infiltrating the bucca, palate and retromolarly the mandible and its metastases. For the reconstruction of the defect involving two surfaces, double plastic procedure was applied with forehaed and BAKAMJIAN cutaneous flaps (1965). The forehead flap was prepared in the traditional way while the Bakamjian deltopectoral flap with laser, respectively. The wound healing was undisturbed.

4.3.2. Endonasal laser operations

4.3.2.1. Operative circumstances

When performing endonasal laser operations the proper exploration and good vision of the operative field as well as the conditions of the laser application must be ensured.

For nasosurgical purposes 25 to 40 W CO_2 laser coupled to operation microscope is used. Accessory equipment includes standard rhinosurgical instruments and a variety of otologic microsurgical instruments. The nasal cavities and choanal regions can be well seen with the microscope by using self-retaining nasal specula or retractors, or by using ear specula of the largest size which fits through the nares. The ear specula has the additional advantage of shielding the alar rim of the nares from the laser beam. The speculum can be manipulated by hand or fixed on a holder. Better illumination for the microscopic vision within the nasal cavity can be readily ensured by a fiberoptic light bundle of a laryngoscope. The tip of the bundle is passed along the edges of the specula. Small-diameter suction tips (Fraser, Barony, or laryngeal microsurgical types) permit suctioning in the cavity without obstructing the vision. Suction is necessary to remove the smoke and steam from the laser vaporization, as well as blood and secretions.

The safety of the patient and the operating team is exceedingly important. The two main hazards can be caused either by the accidental laser irradiation of unprotected tissues or by the fire of inflammable materials.

The general principles of preventing the first hazard have already been described. Nevertheless, there are special tasks to be fulfilled. The patient's eyes must be covered with saline-moistened gauze pads and secured with tapes. The other parts of the face are covered with multilayer moistened gauze. The personnel in the operating team must wear spectacles or safety glasses against the reflected laser radiation. The surgeon must keep his hand outside the path of the beam.

The surgical intervention is performed under general anaesthesia to avoid undesirable movements of the patient. For adults, if possible, metal, flexible endotracheal tube should be used. In children, or adults if necessary red rubber endotracheal tubes are to be applied. The tubes must be wrapped with aluminium tape or other protective materials. Metal connectors must be used.

The patient should be positioned so that his head is at the "foot" of the table. The shoulders are supported by a rolled sheet or thyroid-like cushion. The neck is anteroflexed and the "extended head" lies on a round cushion. The patient and the table are lowered 15° to 20° in the Tendelenburg's position. These details are of utmost significance both for the access of the laser equipment and the physical comfort of the operating physician.

In case of intranasal interventions, after clearing the nose of the secretions, the blood vessels are constricted with 0.125% or 0.25% phenylephrine hydrochloride. A saline-moistened gause sponge is placed in the rhinopharynx to protect this area from the laser beam after removal of the anterior tissue and the orifice of atresia. Within the nasal cavity the laser beam is directed by micromanipulator and aiming light. Towards the choanal atresia, the beam is directed along the nasal floor antero-posteriorly. The nasal floor, the maxillary crest and the turbinate are excellent landmarks for an experienced rhinosurgoen. Permanent suction is essential to remove the occurring steam, smoke and secretions, and to ensure the continuous visibility of the nasal structures.

The hemostatic effect of the laser minimizes the peri- and postoperative bleeding. If seeping occurs and persists, nasal tamponade should be made. For small areas oxidized cellulose pack, for larger ones cots filled with gauze are preferably used. Microfibrillar collagen might be useful for the bleeding of patients with coagulopathy. The tampon can be removed in 24 to 48 hours.

When creating a lumen like e.g. in the correction of the choanal atresia, stents of Silastic or polyethylene tubes are placed to maintain the lumen. The posterior end is cut on a bevel and the tube is placed with the bevel downward. The tube is sutured to the septum with nylon sutures. The stents are kept in this position for four weeks. Humidification, including mist and saline drops, is essential to reduce or prevent crusting. It is necessary to suction the tube lumen several times a day.

Stent plastic intervention is not always needed for other types of rhinologic laser surgery. In case the septum and the lateral nasal wall mucosa have been extensively removed, a silastic sheet is sutured to the septum with a nasal splint in order to avoid the development of synechia. This sheet can be removed after 10 days.

If stent plastics is necessary, the patient is given antibiotics, until the stents are in place. This seems to considerably diminish the formation of granulation tissue around the plastics and most likely the formation of stenosis, too.

4.3.2.2. Correction of choanal atreasia

The first and outstanding application of the laser in rhinologic surgery has been the correction of choanal atresia. This difficult operation can be easily, rapidly and accurately performed by the laser. To approach the operative field transnasally is extremely difficult, especially in children and infants. The procedures described previously have been performed "blindly", therefore they involve certain risks. The microsurgical technique is labour- and time-consuming because the operative field is obscured by bleeding. Laser operation is performed under direct vision; the hemostatic effect of the laser reduces the bleeding. Other structures are not endangered or violated.

In addition to the general surgical techniques described previously numerous further points should be stressed. The laser beam is directed to the choanal atresia along the floor of the nose. Subsequently, this region is vaporized until the protective sponge in the nasopharynx becomes visible. The choana is enlarged to an extent corresponding to the age and development of the patient. In case the atresia consists of a bony plate thicker than 1 mm, the bone is removed with forceps. This prevents excessive heat-conduction from the bone, which may injure the adjacent tissue or produce necrosis or sequestration. Effort should be made to remove as much of the posterior septum as possible.

The results are satisfactory, e.g. out of 11 bilateral and 6 unilateral corrections of choanal atresia in 12 patients no additional surgery was required. In 3 patients secondary intervention had to be performed either on one or both sides.

4.3.2.3. Removal of hemophilic and tumorous tissues

Indications of the endonasal application of the laser are various, e.g. in patients with blood dyscrasia or coagulopathy since they tolerate laser intervention with little or no blood loss. The performance of other techniques is difficult in these cases. Vascular lesions like telangiectasias or small angiomata can be vaporized without considerable loss of blood or without need for skin grafts. Generally no intranasal packs are necessary. It is recommended to remove the anterior nasal lesions in local anesthesia, the posterior ones in narcosis, respectively.

Large masses of intranasal tissue from granulomatous diseases, papillomas or polyps can be vaporized in a short period of time, by using higher power. The septum, turbinates and posterior choanae serve as landmarks and should be preserved.

Occasionally the polyps are removed by microlaryngeal cupshaped forceps. It permits the laser incision of the stalk of the polyps without vaporization, thus the operative time can be shortened and the epithelial tissue preserved.

The patients have none or insignificant postoperative complaints. Bleeding is rare and easy to control by using packs. Local swelling is extremely mild, especially in comparison with that observed following other methods. Patients are often able to smell again, especially after removal of obstructive lesions like polyps. Crusts do develop but can be decreased with saline or glycerol drops or saline douches. Healing is rapid, it takes only a few days for small and two weeks for extensive lesions, respectively.

4.3.3. Complications

According to the literature complications have practically not existed. However, they can occur easily if the principles and techniques described previously are not strictly followed. The excessive application of the laser to a thick plate of the bony part of choanae producing atresia is accompanied by a high heat absorption and subsequent necrosis and sequestration with stenosis.

Raw, non-epithelialized surfaces and circumferential wounds may adhere or contract when healing and synechiae or stenosis may occur. These can be avoided by using stents or silastic splints, and by sparing the skin around the nares. Adequate humidification, the use of suction and saline drops are important to minimize crusting and keep the stent tube open.

4.3.4. Advantages

The most significant advantages of the laser application in rhinosurgery are as follows:

1. Marked hemostasis and reduced blood loss;
2. Minimal edema of the surrounding tissues;
3. Excellent healing;
4. Minimal postoperative discomfort;
5. Applicability to all age groups;
6. Simplification of the surgical technique;
7. Minimal hospitalization;
8. Maximal hospital utilization;
9. Applicability despite coagulopathy or blood dyscrasia.

4.4. Precanceroses and tumours of the lip

Real lip tumours are regarded as those originating from the red part of the labium. They account for 2 to 2.5% of all malignancies. The rate of basal cell carcinomas is 95%. Among them 85% is represented by the keratinizing and 15% by the non-keratinizing and anaplastic forms.

The precanceroses comprise: the glandular cheilitis, exfoliative cheilitis, leukoplakia, leukokeratosis and keratoachantoma. The precancerosis means the cellular atypia and degeneration of the superficial layers of the lip. If the process infiltrates the basal membrane and a malignant cell transformation takes place, "carcinoma in situ" is concerned. In case the tumorous process involves the mucosa as well, it is already the cancer of the lip. The musculature, skin and mucosa of the lips are rapidly infiltrated. According to the TNM-system the T_1 group includes tumours less than 2 cm in diameter, T_2 group those of 2–4 cm, T_3 group includes deep-growing tumours while tumours infiltrating the adjacent organs are classified as T_4. Eighteen per cent of the lip tumours is T_1, 33% T_2, 32% T_3 and 17% T_4, respectively.

More than 200 different types of surgery have been described for the removal of precanceroses and tumours of the lip and for the plastic reconstruction of the resulting defect. The line of incision made for the removal of the tumour is also appropriate for the plastic reconstruction. These two points of view must be considered in case of the laser excisions as well. Consequently, depending on the extent and shape of the tumour, the type of operation should be selected, then the incisions must be made with laser knife. The lip is a hyperemic organ; the laser operations are accompanied by smaller loss of blood and, due to the closure of the lymphatics, the danger of tumorous dissemination is lower. The oncologically correct laser excisions are followed by a tranquil wound healing, the esthetic result is fairly good. The subsequent reconstruction of the defects can be performed with the classical methods.

It would be especially attractive to use the laser for the traditional linear excision or vaporization of the lower lip. From the above oncological points of view, however, this intervention is indicated only for precancerous and in situ carcinomas, the latter completed with interstitial Curie-therapy.

For the operation of T_1 tumours of the lip the wedge resection was widely preferred. Since, however, the lymphatic vessels go from the lip to the submental and prevascular lymph nodes (as first metastatic sites) perpendicularly in the middle third while perpendicularly and laterally in the lateral thirds – it is feasible to perform the excision rather in such a direction that it can include the longest possible part of the lymphatic vessels.

In T_2 and T_3 tumours, the wide quadrate excision is the most reliable method, with the mobilization of the wound edges and simultaneous reconstruction supported by subsidiary incisions.

We recommend the Grimm (including the quadrate excision) or Diffenbach-Bernard operations because they are suitable – by proper selection of incision lines – not only for T_1 but T_2 (2–4 cm in diameter) and T_3 (deep infiltrating) tumours as well, furthermore, they offer favourable plastic surgical results. The T_4 lip tumours involve the bone, therefore their laser removal is discussed in connection with the osseal laser surgery.

In our clinic we performed 6 laser vaporizations with handpiece due to lip precanceroses. Previous probe excision was also made for histological examination. The operation was performed on outpatient basis, under local anesthesia. The vaporization took place in the normal tissues 3 mm from the edges of the lesion, in 2 mm depth. Surgery lasted only for a few minutes. Technical difficulties, bleeding, postoperative complications were not encountered. The wound healing was not prolonged. During the follow-up period of 2.8 years on the average relapses or tumour recurrences could not be observed.

For T_{1-3} cancers of the lower lip we have performed modified DIFFENBACH-BERNARD operations, among them 6 with CO_2 laser (Fig. 17a, b, c). All layers of the lower lip and buccal plates were cut with laser in a way that the assistant, by fingers, pulled the skin adjacent to the incision line to two directions. Thus the incisions could be made relatively rapidly, the duration of operation was not longer than by the use of conventional methods. The wound surfaces were almost dry, allowing to identify the circular arteries of the lip which were cut through between ligatures. Since the line of incision in the Diffenbach-Bernard operation should be made in several directions the use of handpiece caused less difficulties because the spatial mobilization through the articulated system is not really easy and smooth. Similarly to conventional surgery – the wound healing was good and not prolonged. No significant postoperative pain was mentioned by the patients. During a follow-up period of averagely 2.4 years no local recurrence was seen;

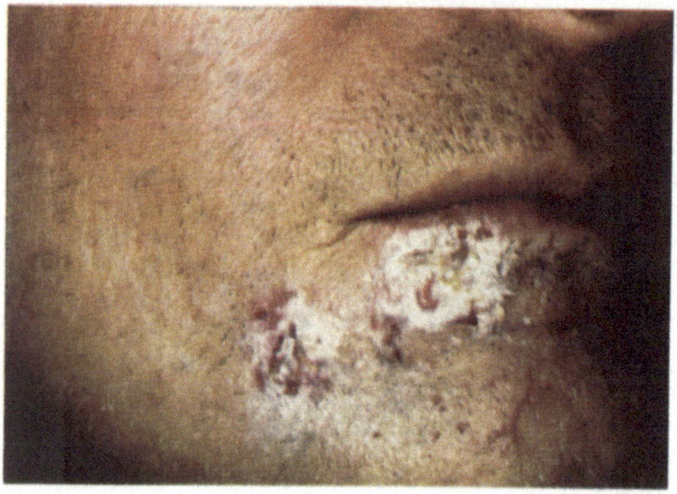

Fig. 17a. Squamous cell carcinoma of the lower lip $T_3N_0M_0$

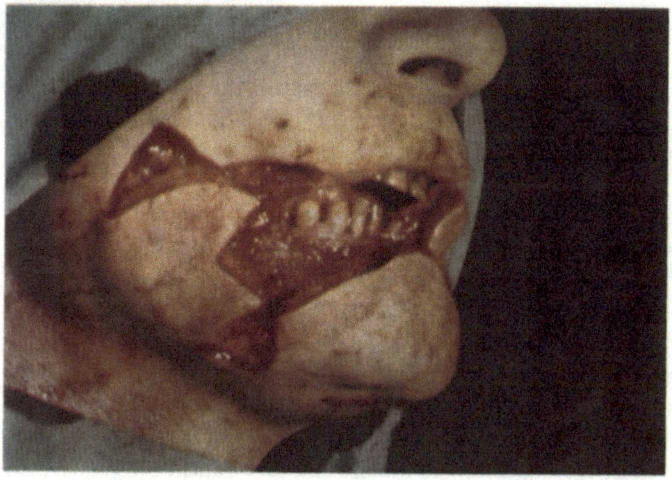

Fig. 17b. Condition after laser excision

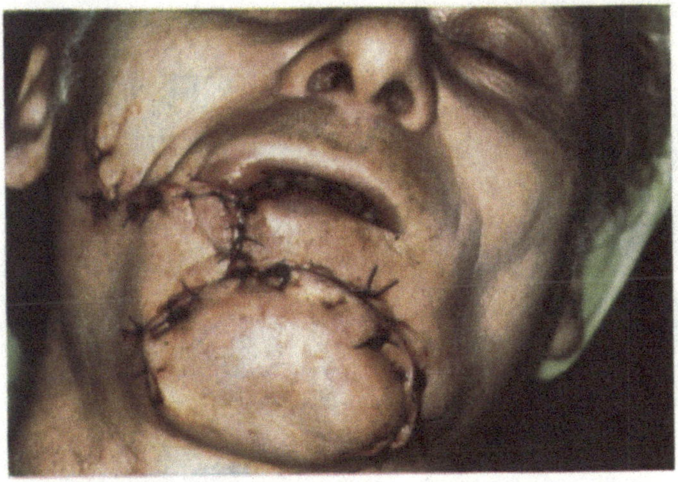

Fig. 17c. Condition after wound closure

regional cervical metastasis developed in 1 patient 9 months following the laser surgery (in this case a secondary RND was performed, the patient has been tumour-free 14 months after the operation).

4.5. Precancerous states and benign tumours of the oral cavity

The overwhelming majority of the precancerous states of the oral cavity is composed of leukoplakias, erythroplasias and papillomas. Among the benign tumours mainly hemangiomas, lymphangiomas and fibromas can be found.

In their therapy the use of the laser is especially indicated (including patients suffering from diseases of the hematopoietic system) because a part of the lesions is hemophilic, and the organs of the oral cavity are hypervascularized. Other advantages of the laser are also predominant.

Due to leukoplakia 8 operations have been performed by the CO_2 laser handpiece in our clinic (Fig. 18a, b). The interventions took place ambulatorily in local anesthesia. The assistants explored the oral cavity lesion, isolated the operative field with moistened gauze pads from the surrounding tissues. By appropriate illumination we vaporized the degenerated mucosa with a continuous laser beam. The operative field remained almost entirely bloodless. The only difficulty was connected with the spatial rotation of the handpiece. Immediately after the operation the patients went home and the next day were able to work. The postoperative pain was minimal and easy to relieve. On the day following surgery the patients could orally consume their usual foods. The operative wound healed perfectly. Scar formation was not observed even when more extended fields were vaporized and the wound was not sutured. No recurrence has been seen.

The literature reports on similar success in the laser treatment of considerably larger patient population, not only in precancerous states but in the so-called "malignant benign tumours" (hemangiomas, lymphangiomas) as well. The laser is excellent for treating planotuberous (superficial) hemangiomas. The duration of surgery, the patient's burden and the quality of wound healing approximately corresponds to those at cryotherapy. Its superiority to cryotherapy as the extent of the surgical destruction can be

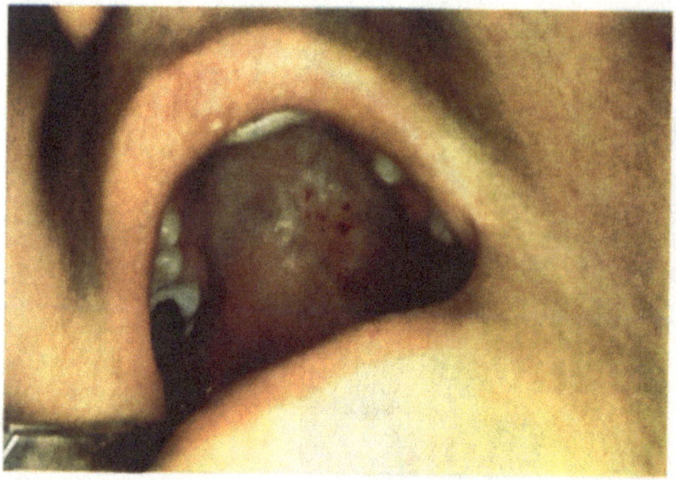

Fig. 18a. Leukoplakia on the roof of the mouth

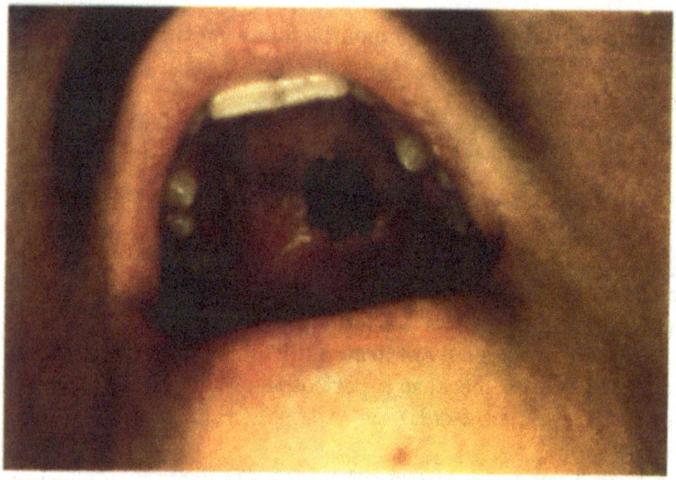

Fig. 18b. Condition after laser evaporization

better controlled, generally only one intervention is needed and the wound healing is more rapid. This relates to hemangiomas infiltrating deeper tissues as well. As an example the treatment of a hemangioma infiltrating originally the nasal mucosa, tongue, floor of the mouth, submandibular region and the neck is reported on. After the conventional procedures applied by several steps (scalpel, electrocauter) the residue involving the tongue was removed by laser. Contrary to the previous operations, after the use of the continuous laser beam the patient could take nourishment perorally on the day of surgery, felt moderate pain, and had an undisturbed postoperative period. The up-to-date treatment of the arterio-venous hemangiomas is the embolization performed during selective angiography with the subsequent surgical removal in a few days. Emboli of different materials injected into the tumour nourishing arteria through the selectively introduced catheter stop or considerably diminish the perfusion, thus the blood perfusion decreases and so do the extent and the hemophilia of the tumour. Frequently – within a few days – sterile necrosis begins. If embolization is not followed by removal of the tumour in some weeks or months, the smaller arteries running to it get dilated, leading again to a greater blood perfusion. If the laser extirpation takes place shortly after embolization, the hemangioma can be radically removed. Since the emboli injected through the main supplying arteries close the lumen of the arteries only at the site of division, the main afferent trunks and the efferent larger veins must be ligated also in case of laser removal. By the use of laser the loss of blood is still significantly less due to the coagulation of the smaller supplying arteries by the laser scalpel. The wound surfaces obtained are suitable for any type of reconstruction. If the hemangioma infiltrates the extracavitary vital organs or, for some reason, the embolization - reconstruction cannot be performed, the sense of palliation is doubtful. The extent and circulatory condition of the hemangioma (i.e. the indication and surgical plan) are precisely demonstrated by the series of angiographic pictures. The laser surgery of the oral cavity can be encumbered by the unfavourable localization of the tumour. These difficulties can be overcome by the endoscopic laser equipment.

4.6. Malignant lingual tumours

Among the oropharyngeal tumours 20% is represented by the lingual cancer extending from the tip of the tongue to the circumvallate papilla. Ninety-nine percent is epithelial cancer (the ratio of keratinizing and non-keratinizing histologic types is 1:1). In 66% of the cases the tumour develops on the edge of the tongue. In case of lingual tumours the surgical application of the laser is especially justified by the fact that at the moment of cutting the laser beam seals the blood and lymphatic vessels to 0.8 mm (Horch, 1977) or to 1.2 mm (Schönberger et al. 1979) or perhaps to 3 mm (Mullins et al. 1968) in diameter, thus the bleeding is small, decreases almost by 90%. The cellular dissemination is minimal. The laser is applied in no-touch way, the operative field is sterile, there is no contamination. The wound healing is excellent and undelayed.

Under experimental conditions Horch (1977) histologically studied the laser-cut surface of the tongue. The necrotic zone was 0.2 to 0.7 mm wide. By the third postoperative day the wound surface is purged and by day 10 to 11 the operative field becomes consolidated to an extent that the sutures can be removed. Compared to the scalpel-cut wound several authors report on a more considerable scarring by the laser. The incorporation of the autograft is undisturbed. Some investigators have observed diminished postoperative pain and superinfection. Others have conflicting opinions, and have experienced prolonged tissue destruction and disturbed wound healing.

We began to apply the high energy CO_2 laser in our clinic in November 1980. For the excision of the $T_1N_0M_0$ (Fig. 19a, b, c), $T_2N_0M_0$ (Fig. 20a, b, d, c) lingual cancer we have used the handpiece of the laser instrument in 14 cases. The operations were performed by local anesthesia. For cutting 40 W continuous CO_2 laser was used. The patient and the personnel in the operating room were wearing spectacles to protect their eyes. In order to avoid the injuries from inadvertent striking of laser beams the operative field was isolated with saline-moistened gauze. After the first incision we held the surface close to the tumour with a museau while taking care of not tugging the tumour itself, then excised it by traction of the normal edge so that the deep base of the wound could be seen. The traction led to the tension of the larger vessels, consequently to a smaller transection, a slower circulation, thus vessels of 2 mm in diameter could be safely coagulated and the larger ones recognized and managed. Cut surfaces remained almost dry, continuous suction of tissue fluid was ensured. Bleeding was minimal. Ablasticity

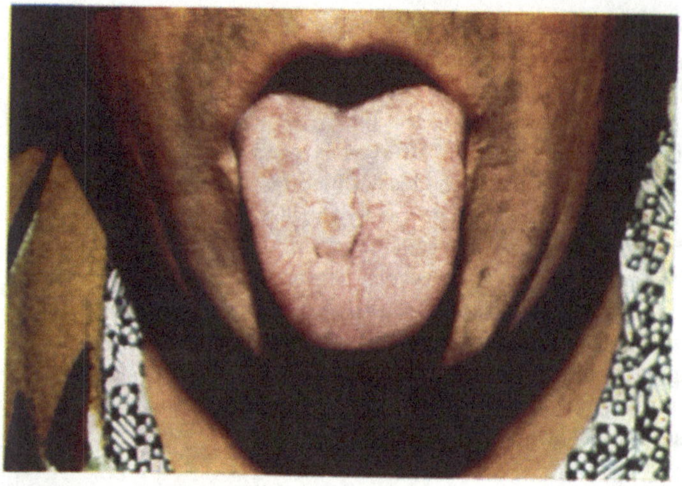

Fig. 19a. Cancer of the tongue $T_1N_0M_0$

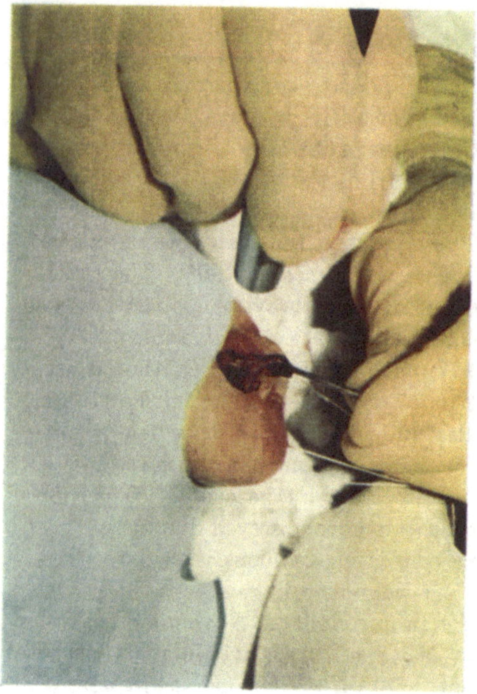

Fig. 19b. Intermediate phase in laser excision

was controlled by intraoperative refrigeration histology, then the wounds were closed with non-absorbing sutures. Since the tumorous process can spread far along the fibres of the lingual muscle tissue in the muscular space and the dissemination can be often prevented by intraoperative probe excision, in case of $T_{1,2}N_0M_0$ tumours surgery was finished by dose-planned radium needle implantation.

We have experienced that the duration of laser operations was similar to that when using electrocauter, and the heat-destructed zone of the wound edges was apparently smaller in the former case. Wound healing was adequate, with the usual extent of

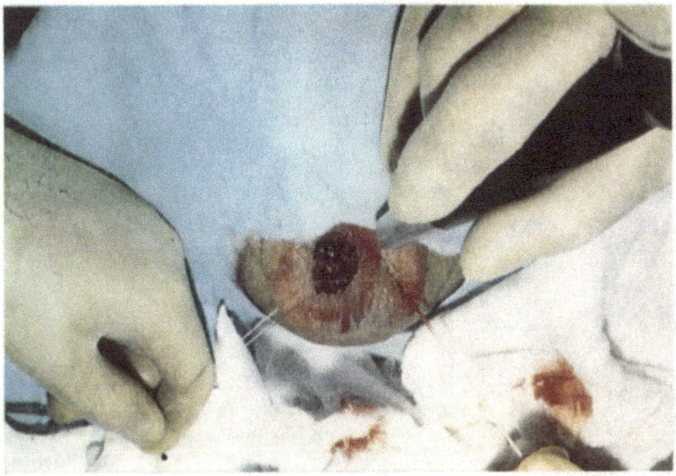

Fig. 19c. Condition after laser excision

scarring. We did not observe delayed wound healing. However, parameters of wound healing are not only dependent on the properties of the laser-cut wound surface, as a consequence of interstitial Curie-therapy, the wound surfaces in the zone of irradiation also suffer more or less radiation damage. Despite the use of radium needles no wound detachment could be seen. Postoperative pain was somewhat milder than usual. Intraoperative tumour cell dissemination could be evaluated only statistically since the occurrence of late regional metastases may result not obviously from intraoperative spreading but from the possible persistence of unpalpable micrometastases at the time of surgery. The histology of our 14 patients is insufficient for statistical analysis.

Tumours of the tip of tongue and those localized on the upper face and side of the anterior third of the tongue are operable by laser without any technical difficulty. These tumours can be well explored, illuminated and isolated, and we operated them on under local anesthesia.

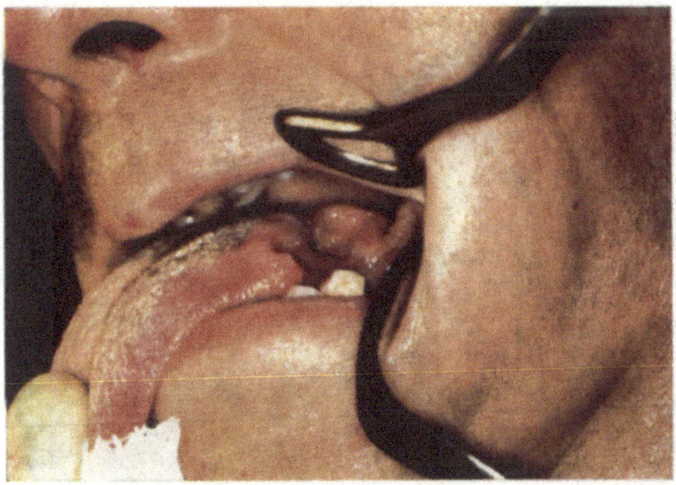

Fig. 20a. Cancer of the tongue $T_2N_0M_0$

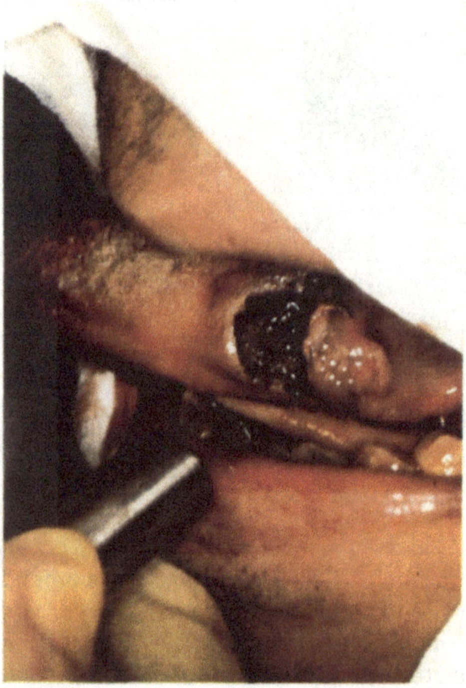

Fig. 20b. Intermediate phase in laser excision

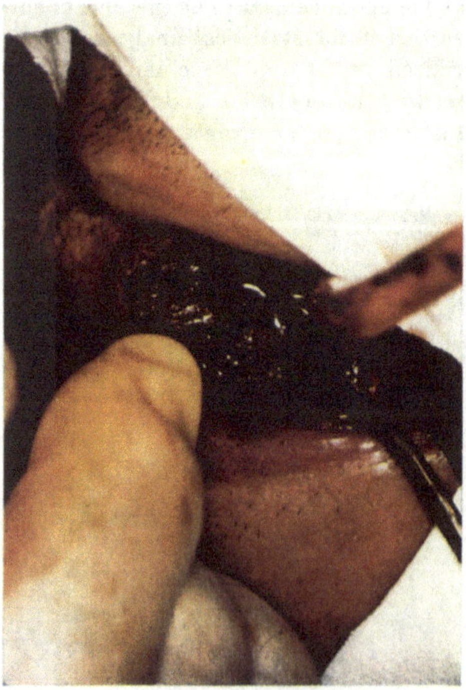

Fig. 20c. Condition after laser excision

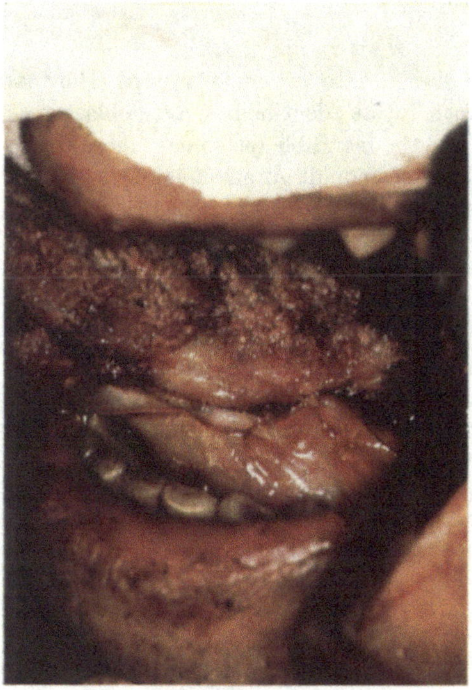

Fig. 20d. Condition after wound closure

Proceeding from the tip to the root of the tongue it gets more and more difficult to use the laser handpiece which should be manipulated in the oral cavity for removal of the tumour. This problem cannot be solved by the endoscopic laser instrument either. It is easier to expose a tumour in the posterior oral cavity by the anterotraction of the tongue. This is associated with pain, besides the possible passage of tumour cells, therefore even T_1 tumours are recommended to be removed under general anesthesia.

If T_1, T_2 lingual cancers have developed regional metastasis into the neck, the monoblock surgery should start with the radical neck dissection (RND). Laser is inadequate for this purpose because it is not suitable for performing the necessary preparations on the cervical vessels and nerves. At the end of the RND the surgical preparation must be pedunculated onto the primary tumour and removed with it in one block in order to remove the majority of efferent lymphatics as well. In case of $T_{1,2}N_{1,2}M_0$ lingual tumours this means a pull-through operation, i.e. the mandible can be saved. After transecting the floor of the mouth the tongue, together with the block, is pulled under the mandible onto the neck, then the tumour is removed. Technically this is the only solution since, due to the mandible, the tumour cannot be passed round from the oral cavity and the neck by the laser handpiece. Following the laser removal of the $T_{1,2}N_{1,2}$ tumours the defects can be closed generally by local plastic procedures. If it is impossible the reconstruction may be made by some myocutaneous flap. Although there is no experience available as yet, it is theoretically presumable (based on the encouraging results of local plastic surgery) that the incorporation of myocutaneous flaps into the laser-induced defects is as good as otherwise.

In case of $T_{3,4}$ tumours of the tongue and floor of the mouth as well as N_3 cervical metastases fixed to the mandible, at radical surgery the mandible should also be resected. These operations are described in connection with osseal surgery.

4.7. Mandibular tumours

The relatively rare manidular tumours can be divided into two major groups. They can be central tumours originating from the tooth (cysts, dentinomas, ameloblastomas, cementomas, odontomas, fibromas, myomas) and the mandible (osteomas, chondromas, osteofibromas, giant cell tumours, hemangiomas, eosinophil granulomas) or peripheral tumours infiltrating the mandible from the surroundings (gingiva, floor of the mouth, etc.).

The management of radioresistant tumours is exclusively surgical task (apart from the eosinophil granuloma responding well to irradiation) while the peripheral tumours can be treated with surgical and radiotherapy.

In the surgery of osseal tumours the CO_2 laser can serve as diagnostic and therapeutic tool. The treatment modality can be selected according to the histological diagnosis. In case of peripheral soft tumours probe excision can be simply performed. If there is any radiological suspicion for bone tumours this is considerably more difficult and can often be done only by special instrument during osteotomy. The intervention may be associated with tissue destruction, marked bleeding and hematogenic tumour cell dissemination. These drawbacks are overcome by the surgical laser.

4.8. Experimental results

In order to investigate the metastasis formation, Oosterhuis et al. (1975) studied the Cloudman S91 melanoma in mice. The melanoma was vaporized with CO_2 laser, and the incidence of local recurrences and pulmonary metastases was compared with that observed by conservative treatment. It was found that the use of laser was not disadvantageous from either points of view.

Since the use of laser is oncologically not contraindicated, prior to its clinical application, certain problems had to be experimentally clarified. For this purpose 12 dogs with 20 to 30 kg of body weight were used. On both of their femurs osteotomy was performed in i.v. Nembutal narcosis. In half of the dogs the first osteotomy was carried out by using 80 W CO_2 laser, in the other half by Gigli's saw. The broken ends were fixed with Allgöwer's 6-hole compression plate for retaining. A few months later, in short narcosis, the healing of the broken ends were controlled by X-ray. Following laser osteotomy two dogs developed osteomyelitis before the sixth month, therefore therapeutic results for only 10 dogs could be compared. After 6 months the animals were used in model experiments on rectal and vocal cord operations. After removal of the plates the high-bones were radiologically examined that time again. Based on the X-ray pictures the animals could be classified into three groups. Complete consolidation was seen after the use of Gigli's saw in 9 and that of laser in 3 animals, respectively. Considering the delayed healing as well, the laser operation results compete with those following conventional transection. In view of all the above it could be established that the healing of laser operated bones was prolonged, consequently the results after using Gigli's saw were superior. This is likely to be in relation with the compression of the broken ends. The stable osteosynthesis of them is a prerequisite of the bone healing. Following conventional osteotomy the cut surface is evenly smooth and the perfectly plain surfaces can be brought into apposition, then fixed by compression plate. On the contrary, laser osteotomy results in a rough cut surface, only certain points of fragments are jointed. (When the laser beam vaporizes the bone, it becomes wedge-like and of uneven surface.) The Allgöwer plate ensures contact and compression only at these points, thus the synthesis is unstable, and the healing of bones is incomplete. In several cases, increased callus formation could be proved by X-ray pictures, the movement of unstable broken ends developed false joints in 2 animals.

In other experiments 26 rabbits, aged 3 to 4 weeks, with a body weight of 800 to 900 g, were examined.

On one limb the distal epiphysis of the femur was excised by laser while conventionally on the other, both in i.v. Nembutal narcosis. The intervention was performed ipsilaterally in 15 animals, and also bilaterally in the others. The power supplied was 7 to 10 E. The animals were sacrificed in week 3 to 16. Each femur operated upon was studied both macro- and microscopically. It could be observed that the central chondric defect between the epiphysis and metaphysis made by laser was filled bridge-like with bone. As a consequence of this growth disturbance occurs on the altered surface, which leads to the shortening of the bone. The bone bridge in the defect exerts pressure on the surrounding tissues. Presumably this can explain the subsequent functional disorder and the slow bone development.

The laser injury of the lateral part of the epiphyseal surface caused growth disturbance on the lateral part of the bone, which led to a valgus-type deformity. Simultaneously, the bone development slowed down.

The bilateral laser injury of the femur resulted in growth disorder, bone shortening on both sides.

Some authors wanted to reveal in rabbits of 2 to 3 kg body weight, under general anesthesia, what are the consequences of osteotomy if performed by drill, continuous laser beam or interrupted extreme energy laser radiation. The tibias of rabbits were transected by the two methods described perviously. Following the usual wound closure and postoperative management the animals were sacrificed in week 2, 4, 8; then the bones operated on were examined roentgenologically and histologically.

The results of investigations are summarized as follows:

1. Osteotomy performed by rotary saw is of longer duration. Laser transection is shorter in time but its effectiveness decreases with depth.
2. Period of healing is somewhat longer following laser osteotomies (confirmed also histologically), the healing process is normal.
3. By the use of laser the medullary bleeding markedly diminishes.
4. Removal of nuisance blood and tissue fluid from the wound surface increases the effectivity of laser.
5. Following both laser methods the wound surface is carbonized. There is no significant difference.
6. Success of the laser osteotomies, after further technical development, may compete with that by using rotary saw, and their routine application can be reckoned with.

Horch (1977), prior to human application, performed osteotomies on the tibias of dogs. The used laser of 34 W or oscillation was with water-cooling. The healing was controlled after the 3rd, 6th, 9th and 12th week by X-ray and histology. Osteosynthesis, with 6-hole compression plate was performed in the first group immediately, whereas in the second one after the mechanical decarbonization of the wound surface. Histological examination made simultaneously with laser osteotomy, revealed the following layers laterally from the line of transection. A 300 micron wide carbonization zone was followed by another 300 micron wide zone from which the osteocytes were missing. In the 700 micron wide third zone residual chromatin was found on the place of osteocytes. In the fourth, intermediate zone concentrically, normal bone tissue can be found. The total width of the 4 zones is 1.3 mm. Three weeks following conventional osteotomy the perichondral and endochondral bone formation is already visible. After laser operation, however, marked antibody reaction and callus formation occurred without decarbonization. In the group of delayed osteosynthesis and mechanical decarbonization a bit prolonged wound healing without antibody reaction was experienced. The 9-week healing period of conventional osteotomies is 12 weeks, both histologically and radiologically, following laser surgery.

The carbonized tissues are supposed to have a stimulating effect on the wound healing, since the healing was evidently delayed in the physically decarbonized group, in comparison with cases in which the synthesis of osteotomic surfaces took place without removal of the carbonizing matter. This is likely to be caused by the fact that following laser surgery the bony substance, osteoblasts and mucopolysaccharide-protein complexes that play a role in the bone formation, get heat-destructed, denaturated. The carbonized bone surface chemically proved to be hydroxyl-apatite originating from the vaporized inorganic bony substance. The hydroxyl-apatite and other carbonized components, through the foreign body reaction and indication of resorption, enable the factors of osteogenesis to induce the bone formation.

4.9. Clinical experiences

After the animal experiments described, Verschueren (1976) introduced the CO_2 laser into orthopedic surgery. One of the first operations was performed on a radiologically diagnosed Ewing sarcoma not extending through the cortex of the bone. The diagnosis was confirmed by isotope examination. Metastasis could not be detected by any method. In intratracheal narcosis the skin, soft tissues and cortex containing the sarcoma were incised by the handpiece of Sharplan 791-3 instrument in a way that the histologic examination following decalcination of the contralateral bony surface verified the radical surgery. After primary wound healing the patient was released from hospital. From animal experiments and clinical experiences acknowledged investigators have drawn the following conclusions:

1. After the use of CO_2 laser the wound healing is delayed but the restitution is not excluded.
2. If oncological causes necessitate atraumatic bone excision the use of laser is advantageous.

According to Horoszowski et al. (1976) the application of the laser can be favourable from other points of view, too. The rate of possible postoperative hematomas, pain, inflammation, superinfection and adhesion can be diminished. The performance of bone surgery by laser can have absolute and relative indications or contraindications.

4.10. Indications

The group of **absolute** indications includes operations on the tumours and hemorrhagic diseases.

Bloodless excision and vaporization of bone tumours resulted in favorable experiences.

In head and neck surgery bone operations are performed if the tumour orginates from the bone or infiltrates it.

Among bone tumours the defects formed after removal of tumours of the hard palate or nasal sinus are not reconstructed with bone grafts. Defects of the skull-cap can be reconstructed with prostheses, that of the nasal bone with bone palate, the resected mandible – which is the most frequent case due to central and peripheral tumours – with free bone transplants, prostheses of osteomyocutaneous flaps, respectively. Stable osteosynthesis is necessary only in the case of mandibular reconstruction performed with bone free graft of osteomyocutaneous flap. Thus the experimentally verified most severe drawbacks of laser surgery such as the delayed wound healing, pseudarthrosis formation or necrosis must be reckoned with only in these cases. This is all the more dangerous since the graft remains completely without blood supply and from the remaining bones new circulation must develop. Apart from the trapezius myocutaneous flap, when applying any of the osteomyocutaneous flaps – the predominant blood supply of the bone and myocutaneous components of the flap is different. At transposition the predominant supply of the bone component ceases. Under such circumstances the unstable synthesis between the laser-incised bone surface and the graft is an exponential source of danger. This danger does not threaten if the mandibular defect is reconstructed by prosthesis. Both experimental and clinical findings justify the use of laser for the resection of any head and neck bone tumours. Exceptions are made for those bulky, advanced T_4 lip and T_3 soft tumours of the oral cavity where osteomyocutaneous flaps are used for reconstruction.

Some authors suggest that the CO_2 laser epiphyseodesis is technically simple and is suitable for the removal or shortening of osteophymas. Correction of congenital or traumatic deformities of the mandibular bone is also successful (HORCH 1977).

According to literature data the laser has improved the therapeutic results in case of **relative** indications as well, and hopefully its routine use is only a question of time. In MOORE's (1972) opinion, in comparison with conventional methods, the surgical laser significantly decreases the operative traumatization, and the wound healing is also better.

The use of laser is favourable if we consider the rapid postoperative mobilization of the patient, the restitution of articulation movement, the considerable decrease in nuisance bleeding, postoperative hematoma and oozing (the latter is of major importance under war-like circumstances). These advantages represent relative indications.

4.11. Laser tonsillectomy

The first evidence of using argon laser of 16 W for tonsillectomy comes from 1984. Surgery was performed under general anesthesia. The tube, in its whole length, was protected from inadvertent laser impaction with metallic wrap and was fixed together with the tongue contralaterally. After protracting the tonsil, longitudinal incision was made on the strained anterior palatal arch. Following dissection of the mucosa the mechanic effect of the special instrument used (raspatorium) and the attached laser heat effect were jointly taken use of. With removing the tonsil, the laser simultaneously coagulates the mechanically protracted tonsillar bed and carbonizes it to the extent and depth required. In 6 patients no bleeding occurred, in further 14 cases it was so minimal that it could be readily ceased. No ligature was needed, secondary bleeding was not encountered. Seven patients complained of painful swallowing postoperatively, 2 of them had temporary earache, too. The wound healed readily and the healing was not delayed.

Tonsillectomy with argon laser is favourable since bleeding is minimal hence intraoperative hemostasis does not cause any trouble. Its disadvantage is the difficulty in exploring the operative field, the space for the surgical procedure is less and general anesthesia is needed. No matter how developed the anesthesiology is, it still has risks and may be accompanied with complications.

Nowadays the number of argon laser tonsillectomies is too small to permit us to decide if the advantages outweigh the disadvantages. Therefore its application in the most frequent type of otorhinolaryngologic operation is an open question as yet.

The CO_2 laser tonsillectomy is performed by the laser instrument attached to operation microscope. To provide visualization in the pharynx, Davis-Crowe mouth gag with slotted tongue blade is applied. The patient is under general anesthesia. Since the endotracheal tube is retracted from the operative field, special tubes and metallic wraps are usually not needed. To clear the steam, the surgical assistant holds the suction tube beside the operative field.

The tonsils are sharply dissected from their fossae. As the mucosa of the anterior pharyngeal arch is incised, the muscle fibres can be easily identified and carefully dissected from the tonsillar capsule without causing them injury. In children, the entire procedure is bloodless. In adults, there are generally some vessels in each fossa which will necessitate coagulation with the CO_2 laser and ebonized hemostats or ligatures. Occasionally, the bleeding is so ample that continuation of the laser treatment is impossible. The blood absorbs the laser energy and obstructs further preparation. Fortunately these cases scarcely occur.

The patients complain of little pain in the immediate postoperative period and are able to swallow and open their mouth with little distress on the evening of surgery. During the recovery period the patient feels no or little pain, at least less than after conventional surgery. After one week of recuperation the pain completely ceases. The eschar of the tonsillar fossa does not slough until two weeks after laser tonsillectomy unlike the experience with the conventional procedure. This is probably because the hemostasis and lymphatic coagulation at the time of injury delays the acute inflammatory response and also other stages of wound healing. It is interesting to note that, of several hundred tonsillectomized patients only two developed late hemorrhage. In both cases it occurred one week following surgery.

The advantages and disadvantages of the CO_2 laser tonsillectomy are similar to those described in conjunction with argon laser the number of the former ones, however, is considerably larger. Thus the use of the CO_2 laser for this purpose is evidently justified among the therapeutic modalities.

4.12. Laser in the laryngosurgery

4.12.1. Introduction

In contrast to some other tumours, the absolute and relative incidence of laryngeal cancers shows an increasing tendency. At present, about 2% of all cancers is represented by laryngeal ones. The male/female ratio is 10:1. Polyps, papillomas, pachydermia and tuberculosis are regarded as precancerous conditions. Histologically, 95% of laryngeal cancers is squamous cell carcinoma. According to localization supraglottic, glottic and subglottic groups can be distinguished.

It is very unfortunate that these tumours are often recognized in advanced stage, therefore the tumour and its regional metastases can be removed only by severely mutilating surgery. Sometimes even these heroic resections and reconstructive procedures are unsuccessful. In view of this, it is a major goal to detect these lesions as early as possible and to apply methods which are fruitful and are associated with minimal or no amputation. The appropriate moment for a successful intervention would be the start of pathologic alteration.

4.12.2. Pathologic bases

4.12.2.1. Inflammations

Of the inflammatory laryngeal disease the localized forms of chronic hyperplasic inflammations are the most suitable for laser therapy. Of the supraglottic forms, in case of the mucosal eversion of Morgagni's ventricle – resulting from chronic irritation – the edema accumulating in the submucosa into the laryngopharyngeal lumen above the vocal cords. The superficial epithelium often undergoes metaplastic transformation. This bilateral process itself, and also due to the limitation of vocal cord motion, will cause respiratory distress. Similar causes are present in the degenerative process of Reincke-edema developing on the ligamentous part of the vocal cord. Localized hyperplasia can mainly be observed in the glottic type of the localized chronic hyperplastic laryngitis. In the epithelium or corium the inflammatory exudate organizes and bulges into the glottis. This is the polyp which forms usually in the anterior third of the vocal cord, sometimes bilaterally. Of the hyperplastic forms in case of pachydermia already the keratosis is predominant. The thickened and keratinizing epithelium deeply invades in the corium, the subepithelium underneath loosens and inflammatory infiltrate accumulates. The keratotic area may ulcerate and becomes similar to the carcinoma. It is detectable principally in the posterior third of the vocal cords, but may develop at any site of the larynx. The papilloma, which can be classified also into the benign tumours of precanceroses, is histologically a papillary epithelial proliferation. Its particular danger is in its possible diffuse position that may cause respiratory distress, its ability to recur and turn malignant is extraordinary.

4.12.2.2. Carcinomatous transformation

Laryngeal carcinomas develop during several years or even decades.

Based on the histological structure the mucosal lesions can be divided into three groups. According to Kleinsasser they are as follows:

1. Keratosis without atypia
2. Keratosis with atypia
3. Carcinoma in situ.

All these stages show typical alteration which can be histologically well classified. Leicher claims that not only the pachyderma but the hyperplastic-chronic form of laryngitis, the papilloma with atypic superficial cells as well belong to the precancerous conditions. It is very essential that in stage III the entire epithelium contains atypic cells but there is no infiltration yet. The infiltration already refers to a tumorous process. First it infiltrates the submucosa, then grows continuously and involves the adjacent tissues. Meanwhile it may break through the wall of smaller, mainly lymphatic vessels hence the tumour cells getting into the lumen may initiate metastatization. Intraoperative manipulation of the tumours may contribute to tumorous dissemination. These hazards are decreased by the use of the high energy CO_2 laser (Strong and Jako 1976, Andrews and Moss 1974).

The extent and stage of the malignant processes can be determined on the basis of the TNM system which may be helpful when establishing a therapeutic plan. Primary tumours are classified into T_{1-4} groups. To sum up it can be stated that only T_1 primary tumours are perhaps suitable for endolaryngeal laser surgery. The T_{2-4} tumours can be only externally operated upon.

4.12.3. Advantages and disadvantages of the use of laser in laryngology

To the effect of the low energy laser beam the tissues warm up, biostimulation takes place which – through unknown mechanism of action – specifically or unspecifically promotes the regeneration of the damaged tissues. In the medium range of energy coagulative necrosis develops, just exceeding the diameter of the laser beam. The coagulative necrosis is superficial, thus very adequate for eliminating the superficial, not deeply-invading lesions. A bit higher, 30 to 50 W energy results in the vaporization of tissues in the way of laser beam, leaving tissue defects on their place. Accordingly, the high-energy laser can be used either for vaporization or cutting.

The laser beam has several important properties making its use in laryngosurgery more attractive than that of the scalpel or electrocauter. Some of them will be stressed here. The operative field remains absolute sterile because the manipulation corresponds to the principle of "no-touch" operation. When the laser is applied in conjunction with an operation microscope, an absolute hit safety is provided. In addition, the edge necrosis of the defect formed is 0.2 mm in diameter, and small lesions can be removed by maximal preservation of normal tissues. This relates also to the depth, since the extent of vaporization depends on the optimal level of energy and the duration of irradiation. As a result of the heat effect on the area surrounding the vaporized tissues, 0.2 mm deep coagulative necrosis develops at the moment of cutting. This necrosis immediately closes the smaller blood and lymphatic vessels of the necrotic zone. This has the great operation technical and oncological benefit that the surgery can be performed on bloodless area and without tumour cell spreading. (The latter could not be confirmed in animal experiments performed by Ehrenberger and Innitzer 1978 and Schenk 1979.) The minimal postoperative edema often makes tracheotomy avoidable.

The disadvantages of the laser derive mainly from the technical difficulties of its application and from economical problems.

With the appearance of the medium-high energy laser medicine has obtained an ideal tool for curing precancerous states while with the high energy laser for curing malignancies, respectively. The advantages cumulate in case of endolaryngeal operations therefore it is not by mistake that this new instrument was introduced into the laryngosurgical practice in the early 70s. Following the favourable experiences it became wide-spread in the most different fields of surgery (Jako and Strong 1973).

4.12.4. Initial steps in the laser laryngosurgery

The idea of dissecting the vocal cords with laser is undoubtedly comes from Jakó and Polányi. Jakó started his experiments in 1965, on cadaveric tissues. He used neodymium laser of 1.06 μm wavelength. Since at this wavelength the laser beam absorption in the tissues is only limited, in order to enhance the effect, he injected 5% cupric sulfate into the tissues. By this method he could produce destruction that could be confirmed histologically, only in case of small lesions. In the middle 60s this laser was used in various investigations, with different parameters, and it was proved that the required tissue alterations could be produced. Marked destruction was observed after the laser treatment of experimentally induced tumours. This gave the idea of trying to apply the laser in tumour surgery. After the CO_2 laser equipment had been constructed by Patel in 1965, Polányi made it suitable for surgical use at 10.6 μm wawelength. Jakó began, in 1967 (in Polányi's laboratory), the CO_2 laser treatment of vocal cords removed from the laryngosurgical specimen. After building the microscopic and endoscopic instruments he proved by experiments on dogs that the focused CO_2 laser beam was suitable for the transection of living tissues. In 1968 he removed singer's nodes from the vocal cords of dogs (JAKÓ 1972). Thus a new method, with a new instrument was introduced to laryngosurgery.

The first patient was operated on, immediately with success at the Otorhinolaryngologic Clinic of the Boston University (STRONG and JAKÓ 1972).

The publication opened up new vistas in surgery that has continuously broadened during the past 10 years. Its significance today is already indisputable, its final place in the medical arsenal will be indicated only by the future.

4.12.5. Extra- and endolaryngeal operations

Laryngeal operations performed with laser can be divided into 2 major groups. The extralaryngeal operations are like the classical ones, with the slight difference that only sharp preparation is made and for this purpose the handpiece of the surgical laser is used.

The endolaryngeal laser surgery is performed under endotracheal anesthesia. The larynx is explored, just like in microlaryngosurgery, by means of Weerda or Kleinsasser laryngoscope (Fig. 21a, b) after placing the patient's neck into hyperextended position for better exploration (Fig. 22). Then, the operation microscope attached to the laser instrument (Fig. 23) is set in and fixed. The red ruby laser head light is directed to the operative field, then the surgery is performed, using high energy beam.

4.12.6. Anesthesiological problems and their solution

The endolaryngeal operations by laser have to be performed under general anesthesia. This involves two problems to be solved.

1. The endotracheal tube fills up a part of the laryngeal vestibule and of the glottis, thus visualization of the operative field and the manipulation are hindered.

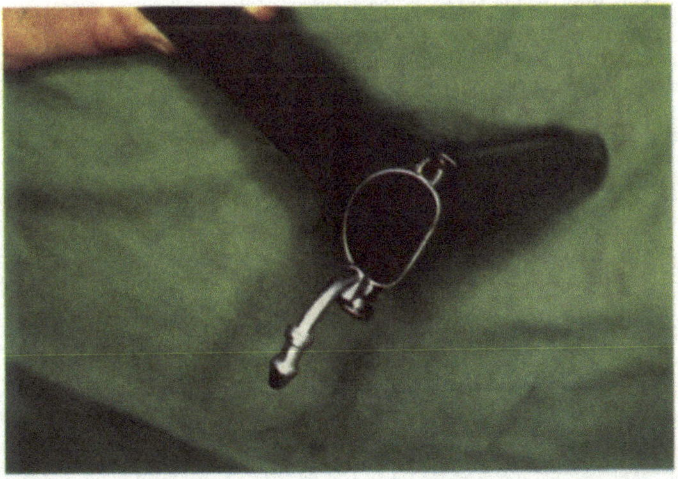

Fig. 21a. Kleinsasser laryngoscope with the fixed smoke-exhauster tube

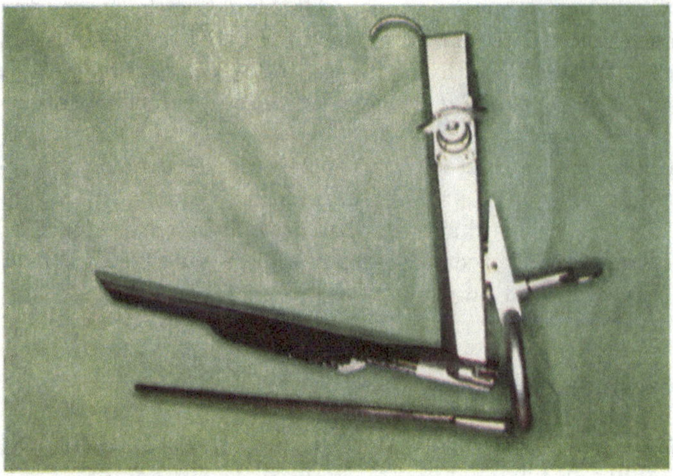

Fig. 21b. Weerda laryngoscope in open state

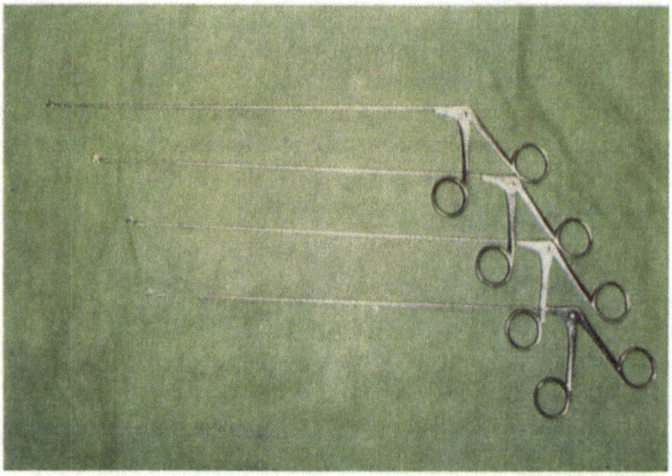

Fig. 21c. Instruments applied for manipulations through the laryngoscope

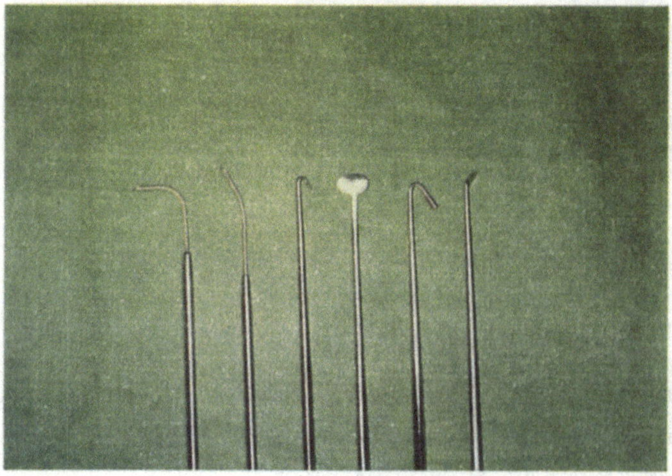

Fig. 21d. Instruments applied for manipulation through the laryngoscope

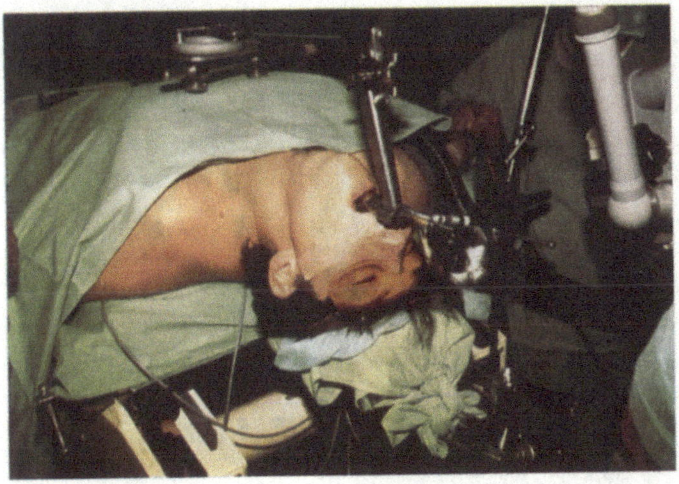

Fig. 22. The patient's positioning for endolaryngeal surgery

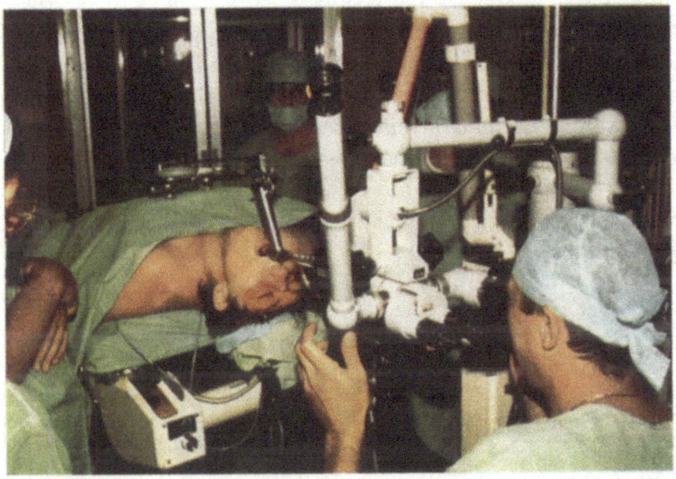

Fig. 23. Setting of the operation microscope for endolaryngeal surgery

2. It is a real danger that by the false direction of the beam the tube gets perforated, the narcotic gas mixture blazes up or goes off, or may perhaps cause unsanitary gas escape.

The first problem can be overcome by using as narrow tube as possible, placing it in the posterior commissure and moving it during surgery. Penetration of the tube can be prevented by using a metal tube (Hirschmann et al. 1980) or a tube with aluminium (Kaeder and Hirschmann 1979) or acrylate (Kumár and Frost 1981) wrap (Fig. 24). A further possibility is the use of injectoflex tube introduced deeply in the trachea. In this case the analgesic gases are passed with overpressure to the tracheal bifurcation through a thin drain. This so-called "jet technique" facilitates both the orientation and operative manipulation. Burian et al. (1981) registered normal blood gas values with jet technique. The expiratory maximal CO_2 concentration measured during narcosis was 4.4 ± 0.4 vol%. Literature data unequivocally show that, when using the jet technique, there is no (artificial) respiratory difficulty in the relaxation phase of the

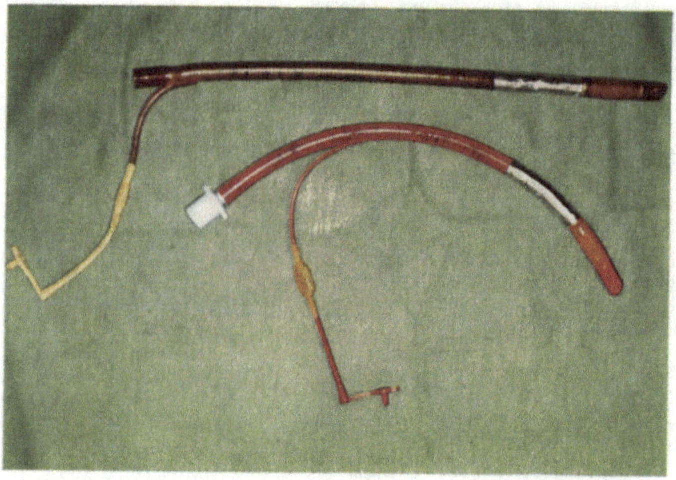

Fig. 24. Tube covered with alfol applied for endolaryngeal surgery

narcosis. According to Krémer et al. (1983) proper selection of the type of narcotic and the concentration of its mixture with O_2 ensures great safety. From this point of view halothene is ideal. The N_2O does not explode either. In case of FiO_2 value of less than 0.3 the explosion risk is inconsiderable. The inadvertent laser beam may injure the surrounding normal tissues, too. To avoid this, the operative field is isolated with saline moistened gauze.

Therefore the tasks of anesthesia are defined by the laser technical requirements of endolaryngeal microsurgery (Krémer et al. 1983):

1. immobile vocal cords
2. reflex protection
3. protection of endotracheal tube
4. corneal protection
5. ideal exploration
6. exclusion of explosion risk
7. intraoperative observation of the patient.

4.12.7. Indications

All lesions treated so far by laryngomicrosurgery are suitable for endolaryngeal laser operation. In addition, it is indicated in all cases when the advantages of the laser described previously may favourably influence the patient's recovery or, if there are certain operative technical advantages by the same expectable therapeutic result.

We started to perform laser surgery in 1980. The type of diseases and the number of patients are enumerated below:

Diagnosis	Number of patients
Benign lesions	
– Morgagni's ventricle eventration	5
– Reincke edema	42
– Polyp	23
– Singer's node	19

Stenoses	
– Laryngeal	9
– Tracheal	6
Precancerous condition	
– Pachyderma	29
– Papillomatoses	16
Dysplasias	
– Cyst	2
– Laryngocele	2
Benign tumours	
– Fibroma	5
– Hemangioma	2
Malignant tumours	
– Supraglottic	
T_{1a}	3
T_{1b}	4
T_2	2
T_3	1
T_4	2
– Glottic	
T_{1a}	102
T_{1b}	10
T_2	6
T_3	4
– Subglottic	
T_{is}	2
T_2	2

4.12.8. Selection of the type of laser surgery

In view of the fact that the hyperplastic inflammations, the keratosis that shows the signs of atypia and the carcinoma in situ are mucosal lesions the laser coagulation of the mucosa and submucosa was assumed to be successful. The carcinoma, however, that is characterized by infiltration, involves the deep-lying tissues as well therefore these tissues must also be removed. In case of T_1 tumour on the free edge of the vocal cord laser chordectomy, in T_1 vocal cord tumour of other site extended chordectomy were the choice of treatment. This spectrum of indication corresponded to a conservative direction. In case of T_{1a-b} cancer of the vocal cord the laser was used for vaporization and not for cutting. For the surgery of laryngeal tumours of other sites the laser handpiece is used as a scalpel. These were classical laryngosurgical procedures where the high energy CO_2 laser beam substituted for the scalpel and electrocauter. From the coagulated or vaporized area a series of specimens were taken for pre-, intra- and postoperative histological examination so that the precancerous or tumorous residue could be removed or the correct choice of the surgical type could be confirmed. The patient was regularly and closely observed even after regeneration of the wound. For T_2 tumours endolaryngeal operations were performed only in exceptional cases. The types of extralaryngeal laser operations are like those with classical interventions.

Since this chapter includes also our own experiences, reference is made to the previous chapters describing the American Coherent 400 CO_2 laser equipment. This can be attached with an OPTON OPMI operation microscope that can be coupled to photo- and film-documentation devices (Fig. 10, 23). The technical conditions of laryngeal laser interventions are improving, at present already complete computerized laser operating rooms are available (Jakó 1983).

4.12.9. Laser surgery of non-malignant epithelial lesions

The causal treatment of chronic inflammations is the removal of hyperplastic mucosa. This was earlier made from thyreotomic incision, nowadays laryngomicrosurgery is performed. The disadvantage of the latter, though more up-to-date method is that, using rigid metal instruments, it is technically very difficult to perfectly remove the mucosa – which is of various shape and extent – and to operate on the edematous, degenerated submucous tissues at an adequate depth. Further source of complications may be the scarring and secondary stenosis following either removal of the mucosa of the anterior commissure or coagulation of the rarely occurring bleeding. These drawbacks or dangers are diminished by the use of the CO_2 laser.

The endolaryngeal CO_2 laser operation is performed under intratracheal anesthesia. The intubation is rarely associated with technical problems since the hyperplastic mucosal degenerations seldom cause considerable luminal stenosis. Occasionally, the eventration of Morgagni's ventricle may be an exception. Intubation, though with smaller tube, can be performed also in these cases, since the edematously loosened mucosa is not rigid. Intubation was followed by the introduction of the Weerda or Kleinsasser laryngoscope, to ensure good visibility of the operative field. Then the tube shielded from the laser beam was set in a way that the entire lesion can be seen and accessible by the straightly directed laser beam. The extraoperative normal surfaces were protected with saline moistened gauze (Fig. 25a, b), thereafter the removal of the lesion started. In case of eventration of Morgagni's ventricle the epiglottis was elevated by laryngoscope towards the root of the tongue, and the edematous mucosa and submucosa getting into sight were vaporized, going towards the vocal cords. Layers under the submucosa were saved. If all or a part of the vocal cords had also been edematous, vaporization was continued on these areas. In case of a partial vocal cord involvement the operation was completed, however, when the whole surface of the vocal cord was inflammatory, it was vaporized only at certain points. The mucosa of the anterior commissure was preserved in each case, in order to prevent the development of synechia. The complete removal of the loose, edematous mucosa was facilitated if the hidden or hardly accessible mucosa was moved in the way of laser beam, by excisors or other instruments. In case of Reincke edema the laryngoscope is directed deeper so that only the vocal cords and some of the vestibular folds get into sight. From the surface of the vocal ligament the loosened mucosa was evaporized. Care was taken to save the mucosa of the anterior commissure (Fig. 25b, 26).

Technically the same procedure should be followed also in case of pachyderma. Since this lesion often develops on the posterior mucosal surfaces, it is necessary – in addition to changing the intraoperative position of the tube – to move the keratotic surfaces, by excisors, into the field of vision. Since the pachyderma was also regarded as precancerosis, the mucosa of the anterior commissure was evaporized, if found necessary (Fig. 27a, b).

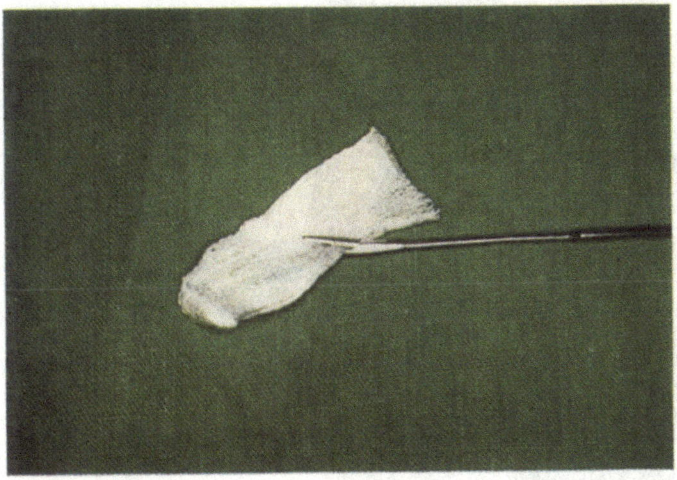

Fig. 25a. Bringing the protecting gauze sheet into the right position by laryngomicrosurgery instrument

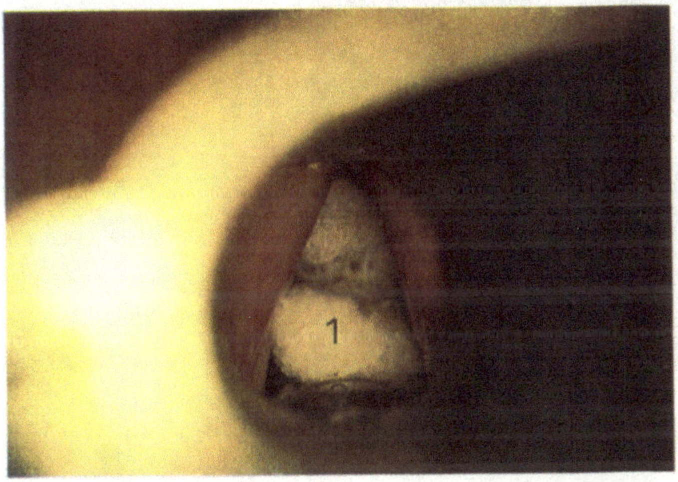

Fig. 25b. Positioning of the protecting gauze sheet in endolaryngeal surgery, Reincke-edema
1. the subglottic placed gauze sheet, 2. tube covered with alfol

For the removal of polyps the laser was applied in two different ways. If the polyp was located on a thin base, it was elevated from the surface and was dissected by laser beam at the mucosal level (Fig. 28).

In case of polyps, singer's nodules and papillomas sitting on a wide base, the laser beam was directed onto the lesion that was evaporized deeply (Fig. 29a, b, c). In case of papillomas we penetrated to the muscles.

In recurrent papillomatosis first the nasal cavity and pharyngeal papillomas were removed, this was followed by the management of the larynx (Fig. 30a, b):

The epiglottis was turned, by accessory instruments, towards the root of the tounge, then the papillomas were vaporized to the perichondrium. Subsequently, one half of the larynx was made visible. First papillomas of the supraglottic area were removed to the

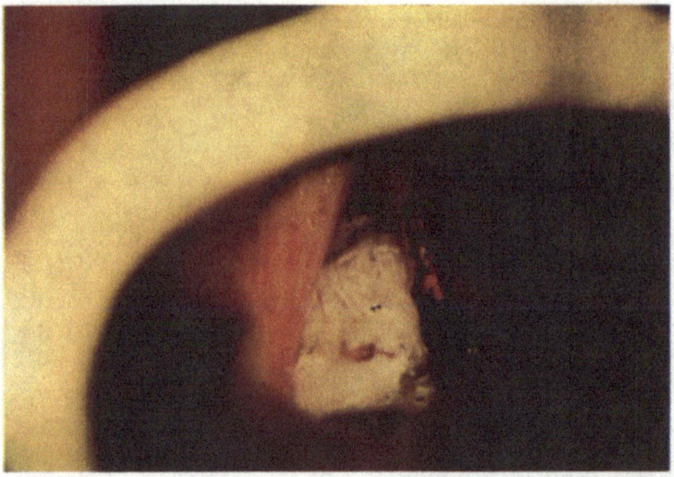

Fig. 26. Reincke-edema after laser evaporation

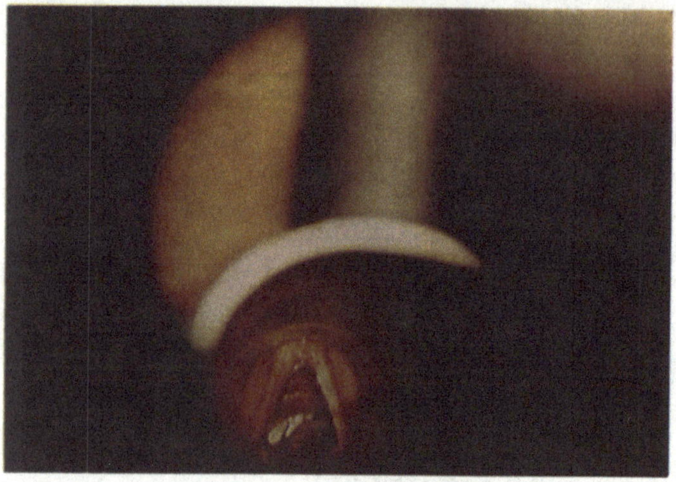

Fig. 27a. Vocal cord pachyderma before surgery

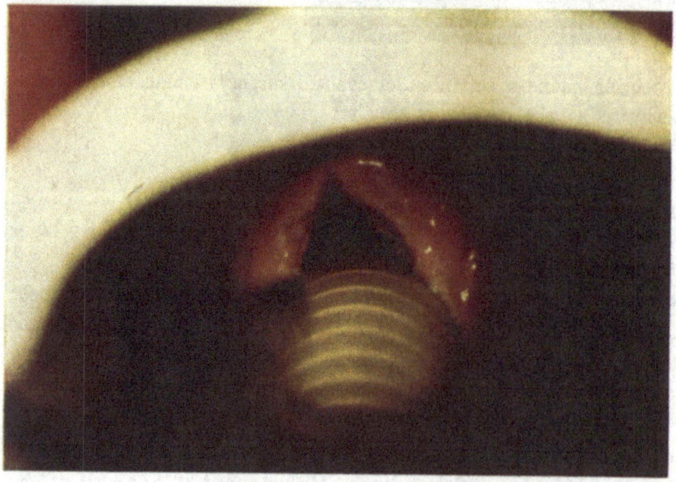

Fig. 27b. Vocal cord pachyderma after laser vaporization

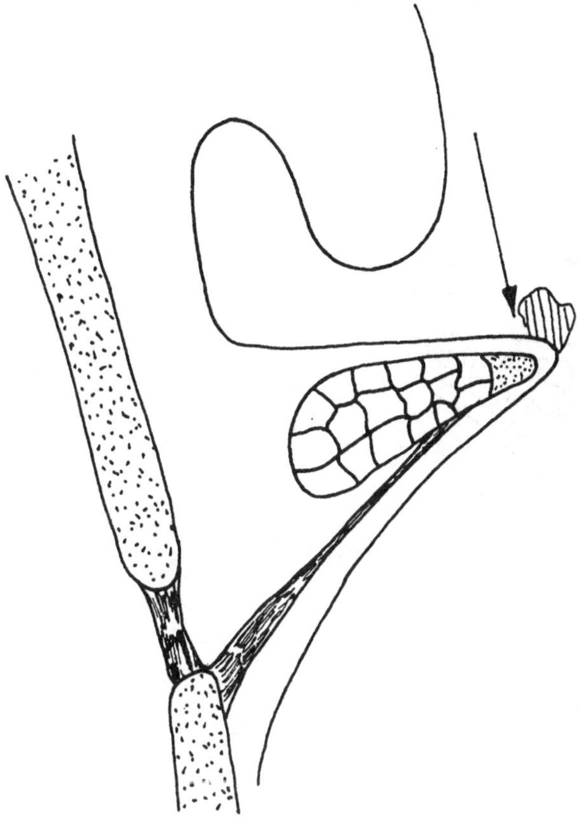

Fig. 28. Scheme of laser excision of vocal cord polyp

muscles, then those located on the vocal cords and subglottic mucosa. In case of multiple papillomatosis of both vocal cords, to prevent adhesion and secondary synechia, it is advisable to lase in the first session only one of them with the anterior commissure. After 6 to 8 weeks, following reepithelization of the lased vocal cord, the other one can also be operated upon without risk. Although postoperative edema is minimal – following extensive laser surgery – to avoid the need for tracheotomy, intravenous administration of antiphlogistics is justified. According to Strong et al. (1976) steroids given i.v., preoperatively (it is not necessary in case of few papillomas) minimize the danger of suffocation – even after extensive interventions. (E.g., out of 210 patients of other authors only two tracheotomies were indicated.) Papillomas under the subglottic field can be operated on by using special equipment (laser instrument coupled with ventillation bronchoscope). Those localizations are excluded where the papilloma is located in the secondary bronchi or pulmonary tissues. Occasional edema following laser irradiation of the lower air passages does not cause severe respiratory distress.

4.12.9.1. Surgical experiences

In all cases the non-malignant epithelial lesions could be made accessible by laser, though by means of appliances. The CO_2 laser beam of 25 to 30 W, by 0.5 to 1 sec interrupted

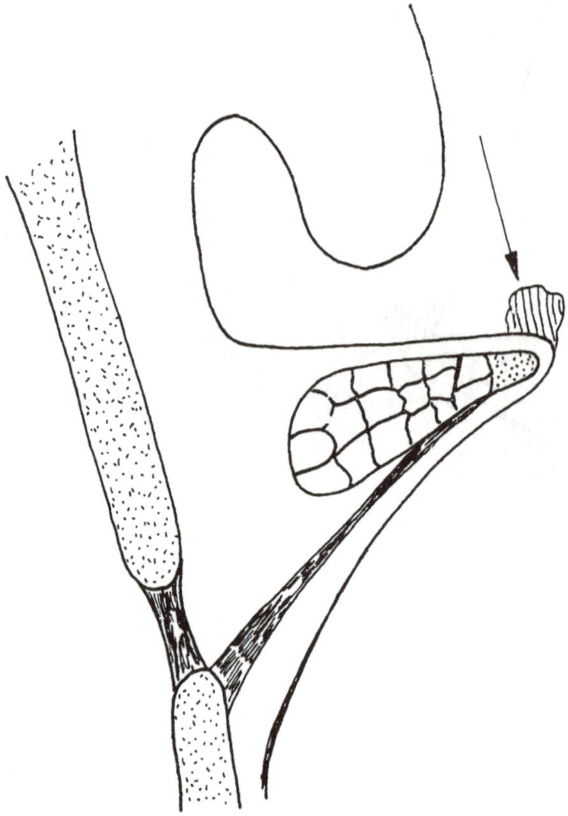

Fig. 29a. Scheme of laser vaporization of vocal cord polyp

Fig. 29b. Vocal cord polyp before laser vaporization

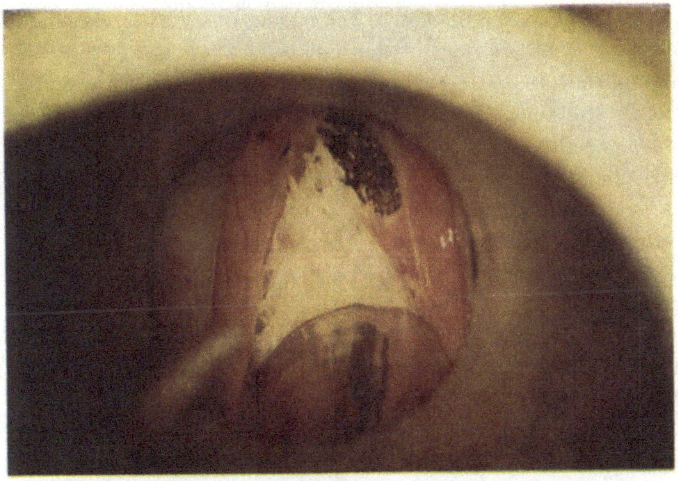
Fig. 29c. Vocal cord polyp after laser vaporization

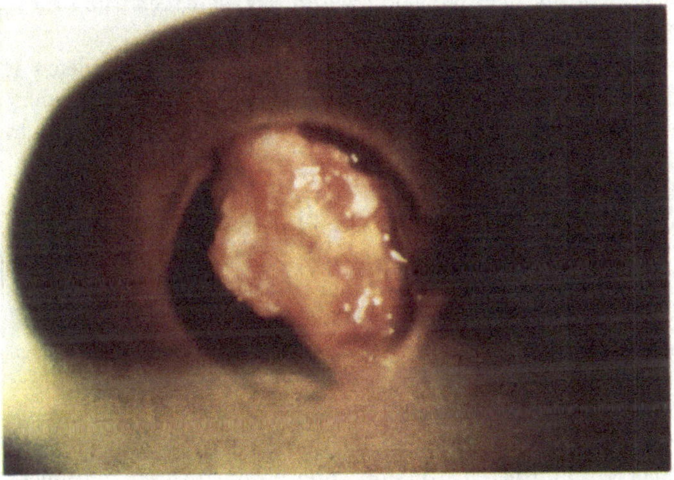
Fig. 30a. Laryngeal papillomatosis before laser surgery

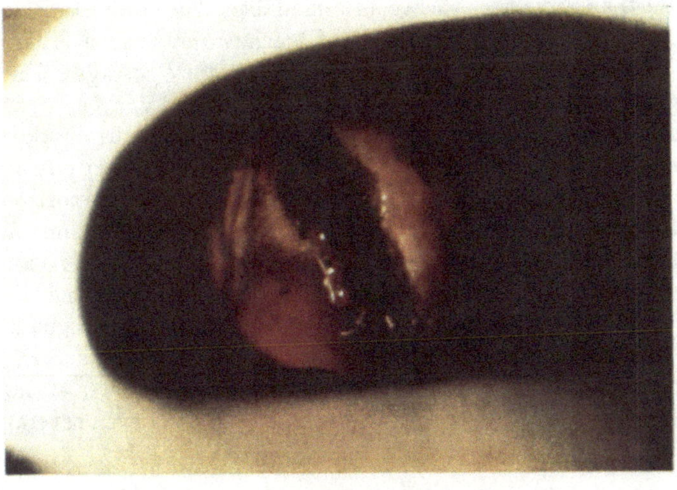
Fig. 30b. Laryngeal papillomatosis after laser surgery

operation, was extremely suitable for the coagulation of the edematously loosened mucosa. When shooting at a point the thermal damage of the mucosa is about 1.5 to 2 mm in width and it extends to the submucosa. After shooting, the "pilot" light is directed onto the adjacent area, prior to another shooting. In these cases the interrupted laser beam is advantageous because the direction of the beam can be set in a way that a narrow stripe remains between the coagulated areas, allowing the start of epithelization. A further advantage compared to the continuous laser beam is that we need not be afraid of damaging undesirable deep structures.

In case of polyps, singer's nodules, pachydermas and papillomas the continuous laser beam is superior, great care should be taken of leading it to the adequate direction and depth, or keeping it at one point. At continuous operation permanent suction of the resultant steam is especially important, to ensure good visibility. The steam of about 100°C may cause thermal damage on the surrounding normal organs.

As a consequence of the simple operative technique the duration of laser surgery is shorter than that of the conventional laryngomicrosurgery, about 15–20 minutes after the onset of narcosis. The hardly accessible areas can also be taken to the visual field, by using special devices. The operative field is bloodless and dry, so-called "nuisance" bleeding was not observed even in case of papillomas.

Following laser surgery – even after coagulation of extended surfaces – the edema is minimal. Respiratory distress did not develop even after removal of multiple papillomas. In this latter case severe respiratory distress necessitating tracheotomy does not seem to occur even without the administration of antiphlogistics.

The reepithelization of the lasered areas takes about 7 days. The patients are allowed to speak, nourish immediately after awaking. On the second postoperative day the are discharged from hospital. The wound-healing is adequate. Scar-formation causing stenosis was not seen. Of 210 patients operated on by other investigators for papillomas only 9 developed adhesion – after bilateral papilloma-removal performed in one session – in the anterior commissure at 2 cm (due to deep excision) on the interarytenoid area. Although in each patient with papilloma recurrence was observed, in the half of them about 0.5 to 1-year symptom-free interval could be achieved. Our own experiences are identical with this. There are literature data suggesting that, following laser surgery, the rate of recurrent papillomas is diminished if adjuvant Interferon treatment is applied. BURIAN's report (1981) deserves special mention, i.e. the laser treatment of childhood papillomas is more successful than any other therapeutic modality. The complete lack of postoperative edema allows to fail the performance of tracheotomy, which is not indifferent from the point of view of the developing upper respiratory passages. The postoperative scarring is significantly less, consequently the movement of vocal cords is undisturbed, the phonation is intact. Following conventional surgery and irradiation extensive adhesions may develop, which necessitates the performance of another operation. This danger is rarely encountered by the use of laser. Though the laser vaporization of papillomas is not a definitive therapy, it can virtually be repeated in an unlimited number, it is technically simple and is associated with no complications. Remission can be achieved with it, it is not mutilating, hence it is the most successful choice among the therapies available at present. Following the laser treatment of the other, non-malignant epithelial lesions the rate of recurrences is minimal. This clinical experience is in accordance with the negative histologic result of the specimen taken from the lasered area at the end of surgery. If recurrence develops the laser operation can be repeated even several times.

4.12.9.2. Benign tumours, developmental abnormalities

Two-thirds of all laryngeal tumours are benign lesions, if the papilloma is also included. Of the benign tumours only those of soft tissue origin are suitable for endolaryngeal surgery. The chondromas, chondrosarcomas can be removed from extralaryngeal incision, with laryngeal resection. The type of resection is determined by the site and extent of the tumours (see e.g. operations of laryngeal tumours).

The fibroma which sits on a wide base of peduncle and originates in the submucosa, has similar manifestation as the polyp. It is mainly of supraglottic location. The histologically mixed forms (angio-, lipo-, neuro-, myxofibromas) are rare, just like the laryngeal epulis, the pseudotumours, the myoma, the hemangioma, the plasmocytoma, etc. The laryngeal cysts and laryngocele are mentioned here because of their similar clinical symptoms and similar treatment.

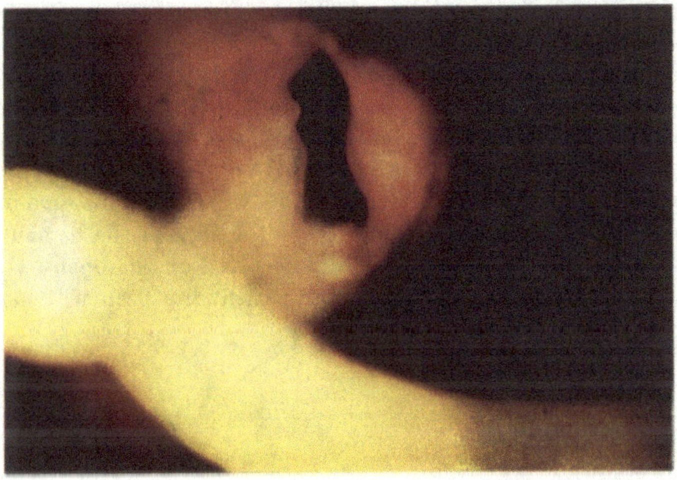

Fig. 31a. Laryngocele of small size before laser surgery

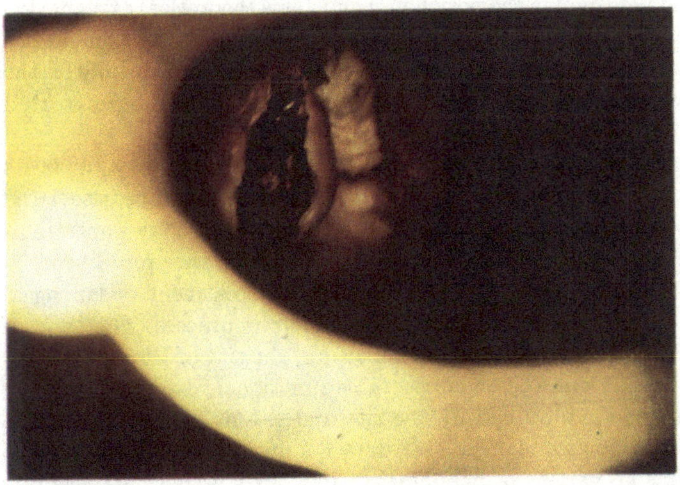

Fig. 31b. Laryngocele of small size after laser surgery

The histological examination plays an important role also in the diagnosis of benign tumours and developmental abnormalities. In our clinic preference is given to the preoperative histology but the intraoperative frozen technique is also accepted. The syndrome and clinical manifestation of the non-malignant epithelial lesions, the benign tumours and developmental abnormalities frequently resemble. The result of the histo-. logical examination is very important because it determines the depth of laser excision. E.g., in case of benign soft tissue tumours the submucosa must be removed in its whole depth. In case of cysts – in order to avoid recurrences – the mucosa forming the interior wall of the cyst must be completely removed. In small laryngocele complete removal is necessary to the neck of the cele – the larger ones are operable only from extralaryngeal incision. In these cases the exploration of the operative field, the application of the laser beam and the results obtained are very similar to those experienced in the non-malignant epithelial lesions.

Because of the extreme bleeding the hemangioma is judged differently. In the therapy of these "malignant benign tumours" the vascular coagulation effect of the laser can be excellently taken use of. Endolaryngeal operation can be performed even in those cases where the angioma is extended and the conventional procedure would be only extralaryngeal. Burian et al. (1981) recommends first to diminish the tumour bulk, using low-power beam, then – depending on the extent, shape and site of the tumour – to perform excision or vaporization. In our clinic we operated on one patient, due to laryngeal hemangioma. During surgery, with 40 W power, we vaporized the tumour without prior debulking. We started vaporization ringwise at the edge of the hemangioma, then proceded towards the centre. Bleeding hardly occurred on the operative field, no tracheotomy became necessary. Since surgery the patient has been without complaints.

4.12.10. Laryngeal cancer

According to Jakó, the endolaryngeal use of the CO_2 laser has made possible not only the removal of certain parts of the vocal cords but also that of bulky tumours provided that the deep infiltration did not involve the perichondrium. This theoretical explanation causes difficulties from the practical point of view since at present there is no diagnostic technique available that could unequivocally detect the tumorous infiltration of the perichondrium. This especially refers to those tumours that had already been treated by other methods.

Another drawback is that the laser beam led to the perichondrium may cause its thermal damage. Thus, inflammation or necrosis may develop, which can be associated with not only complaints, complications, therapeutic difficulties but may contraindicate the postoperative irradiation absolutely necessary after the laser surgery of T_2 tumours. The hesitation concerning the indication of surgical treatment of laryngeal cancers is not only due to the advanced stage of the tumorous process. The type of surgery is also influenced by the organogenesis of the larynx, the site of the tumour, its histologic type, oncological behaviour and the expectable functional result. In the laser operations the classical methods determined by the site and extent of the tumour are most important since the introduction of the laser does not justify the elaboration of new types of surgery (there is no variety of possibilities anyway). Furthermore, the role of the laser is not else than the favourable replacement of the conventional sharp instruments. The decision about the type of surgery also determines the extra- or intralaryngeal use of the laser. In view of all the above, the laser surgery of supraglottic, glottic and subglottic tumours are discussed separately.

4.12.10.1. Supraglottic tumours

In the treatment of supraglottic laryngeal cancer we follow a conservative practice in our clinic. Based on the TNM classification the solutions listed below are chosen:

T_{is}, T_{1a} suprahyoid laryngeal surface of the epiglottis –
supraglottic horizontal resection
aryepiglottic fold –
hemilaryngectomy of supraglottic horizontal resection
Morgagni's ventricle or vestibular fold –
hemilaryngectomy
or in all the 4 localizations – irradiation

T_{1b} laryngeal surface of the epiglottis or on the vestibular fold –
3/4 resection
laryngeal surface of the epiglottis + Morgagni's ventricle –
laryngectomy or "near" total laryngectomy
or in both cases irradiation

T_2 laryngeal surface of the epiglottis + vestibular fold – Morgagni's ventricle – vocal cord
laryngectomy or "near" total laryngectomy"
vestibular fold or Morgagni's ventricle – vocal cord –
hemilaryngectomy (open)
or in both cases irradiation

T_3 laryngectomy

T_4 extensive laryngectomy (resection of the root of the tongue, hypopharyngeal, skin resection) and postoperative irradiation

N_1N_2 radical neck dissection (RND) (in monoblock)

N_3 palliative irradiation and/or cytostatic treatment

Our therapeutic decisions show that the endolaryngeal laser operation has no place at all in our practice. This relates even to the T_{1a} tumours (not reaching the junction of the three cords) on the laryngeal surface of the epiglottis (Fig. 32a, b). The classical surgery of these tumours is the epiglottectomy or the horizontal laryngeal resection. The already outdated epiglottectomy would although be suitable for endolaryngeal surgery, the horizontal laryngeal resection (Fig. 33a) must be performed extralaryngeally. Since the mucosa of the epiglottis is in the direct vicinity of the perichondrium, with a positive histologic finding, the tumorous infiltration of the cartilage must be reckoned with. The radicality of epiglottectomy or vaporization of the tumour located on the laryngeal surface of the epiglottis can be queried. In case of T_{1a-b} tumours of other sites the horizontal laryngeal resection or an even more extensive resection is necessitated by the chondral infiltration and the direction of the tumorous dissemination (Fig. 32a, b). This relates also to the $T_{2,3,4}$ tumours. In our clinic palliative endolaryngeal laser surgery was performed only if the patient refused the conventional operation or irradiation. If the patient neglected surgery only, the laser operation was completed with radiotherapy.

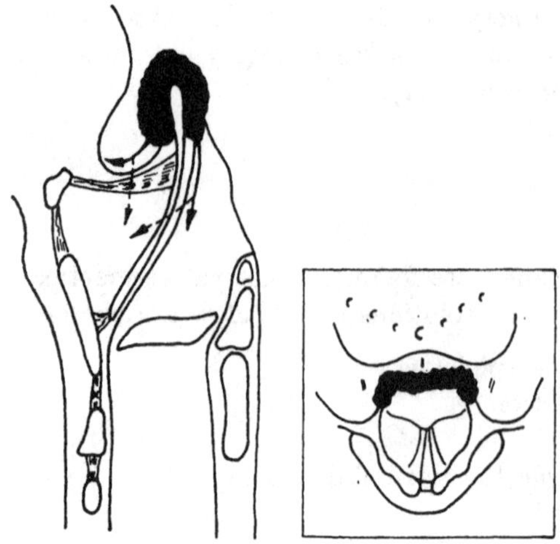

Fig. 32a. The pathways of the supraglottic tumour

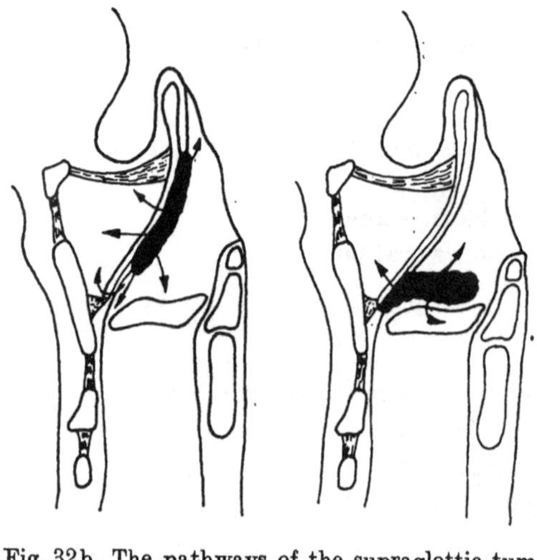

Fig. 32b. The pathways of the supraglottic tumour

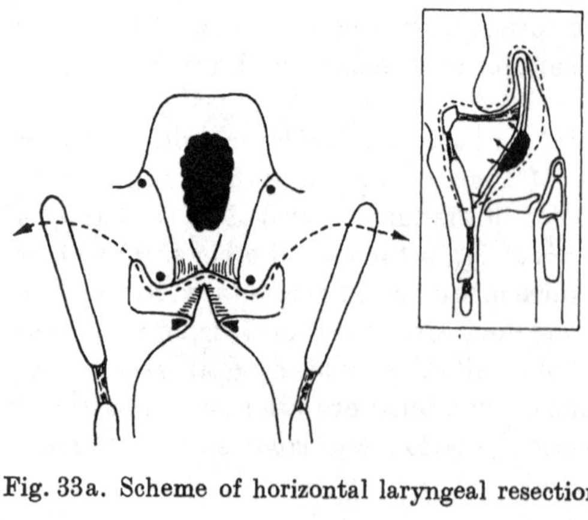

Fig. 33a. Scheme of horizontal laryngeal resection

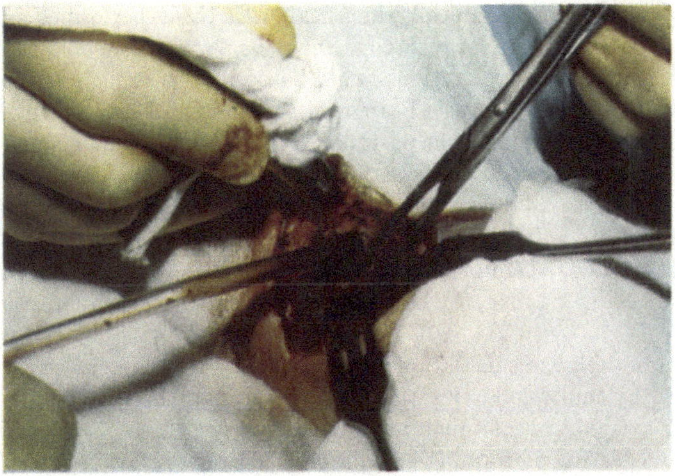

Fig. 33b. Extralaryngeal horizontal resection of the larynx by laser; cutting of the muscles above the hyoid bone, its lifting ahead

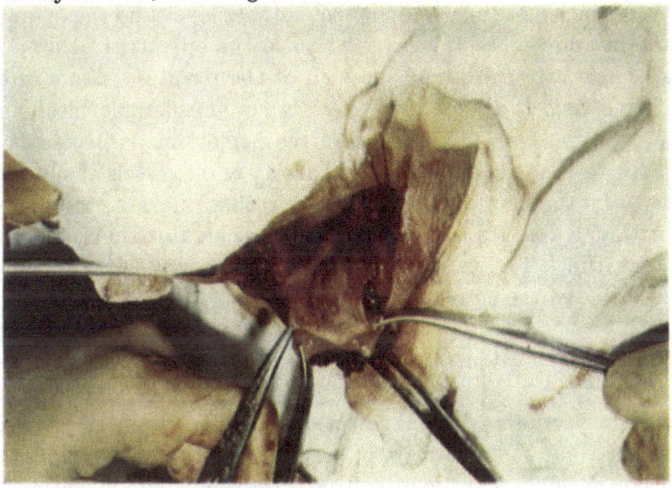

Fig. 33c. Lifting of the epiglottis

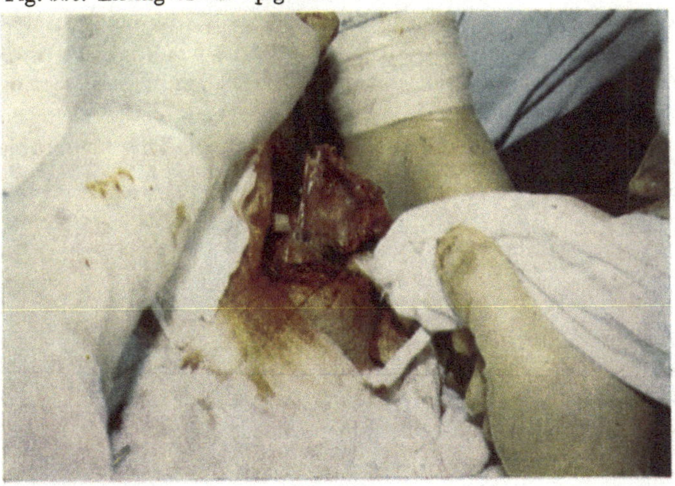

Fig. 33d. Removal of the epiglottis "en bloque" with the hyoid bone and preepiglottic fold

The supraglottic laser operations are technically identical with those performed in case of benign supraglottic processes. The laryngoscope must be carefully introduced into the laryngeal vestibule, so that the exploration should be perfect without injuring the tumour and passing the tumour cells. The laser beam is directed only to the perichondrium. The intraoperative bleeding is minimal, the postoperative edema is small. Tracheotomy is not necessary. The chance of recovery considerably increases with the possibility of postoperative irradiation. Ten to 14 days following consolidation of the operative field the irradiation can be initiated. The scar formation of the operative field is minimal – there is tumour on the surface – therefore the success of irradiation is not reduced for radiobiological reasons. At the same time, the laser surgery can significantly diminish the tumour mass.

If the patient refuses irradiation, the suffocation or tracheotomy can be delayed by several months or prevented by multiple laser surgery. In these cases the patient dies of the consequences of the extralaryngeal tumorous dissemination.

The laser handpiece is suitable for performing extralaryngeal laser operation of any type. The handpiece is used as a scalpel, all the tissues are dissected with it. When cutting through the soft tissues it is feasible to keep the wound edges laterally strained, since the coagulation necrosis of the edges thus extends to a thinner layer and the operation is faster. The assistants – in addition to the exploration of the operative field and traction of the wound edges – ensure the continuous suction of the resultant steam and body fluids. Thus, the operative field is almost dry, there is no considerable bleeding either from the subcutis or the muscles. No intraoperative hemostasis is necessary. Ligature must be performed only on the superior laryngeal artery or on vessels of similar luminal wideness. The spatial movability of the handpiece is rather difficult, therefore a part of the time gained with the absence of hemostasis, is lost. A further operative technical disadvantage is that the laser beam is suitable only for cutting, the preparation in the layers is impossible in the conventional way. For this reason either conventional instruments are used for the assistant pulls the layer margins prependicularly with the line of laser incision. The reconstruction of the wound is performed conventionally.

Though the number of laser horizontal laryngeal resections, hemilaryngectomies and laryngectomies performed in our clinic is low, we are of the opinion that the subsequent wound healing and its quality do not significantly differ from those following conventional surgery. In these cases the oncological advantage of the laser can be reckoned with. The technical drawback caused by the tardy use of the handpiece is hardly compensated by the bloodless operative field. Till the entire wound healing a nasogastric tube must be introduced to the patient and tracheotomy must be performed. The minimal scarring following laser surgery allows us to hope for a small scarry dislocation of the laryngeal stump, thus the swallowing function will sooner become satisfactory. This favourable result has not been seen in the small number of our patients.

4.12.10.2. Glottic tumours

In our clinic the following therapy is applied in the glottic laryngeal tumours:

T_{is}, T_{1a} irradiation or chordectomy
T_{1b} irradiation or partial resection (frontal anterior)
T_2 extended chordectomy, hemilaryngectomy (open, closed) irradiation
T_3 laryngectomy

T_4	extended laryngectomy with hypopharyngeal resection, skin resection and postoperative irradiation in operable cases: palliative irradiation and/or cytostatic treatment
N_1N_2	RND in monoblock
N_3	palliative irradiation and/or cytostatic treatment

The glottic tumours can be firmly differentiated by the TNM classification (Fig. 34), thus the indications are easy to determine. The classical operation of the T_{1a} vocal cord cancer is the chordectomy performed from laryngofission (Fig. 35a). Radiotherapy is an alternative choice. The feasibility of endolaryngeal laser surgery in the T_{1a-3} vocal cord cancers is confirmed not only by the operative technical advantages but the low rate of early complications and recurrences as well (Höfler and Burian 1981). In case of T_{1a} vocal cord tumours the chordectomy is performed by laser endolaryngeally (Fig. 35b). Prior to indicating chordectomy precise topic and histological diagnosis should be available. In case of laser chordectomy the usual procedure consists of the intraoperative excision and histological examination of the lesion, then in case of positivity chordectomy follows. In our clinic the histological and chordofiberoscopic examination are done preoperatively, the intraoperative histology is reserved for conducting the ablasticity of chordectomy.

Some investigators are of the opinion that, using laser, only the extent of absorption thermal damage can be judged, that of the conduction not. Consequently, to avoid complications, the laser chordectomy is felt justified only in case of carcinoma in situ. Therefore also in the T_{1a} vocal cord cancer the classical intervention is given preference. Considering that using the CO_2 laser, the necrotic zone is minimal, its width is known, the conduction thermal damage is also minimal, we support most of the literature data stating that in case of the T_{1a} vocal cord cancer the performance of the CO_2 laser chordectomy is justified and indicated. Although the circle of laser operative indications of the

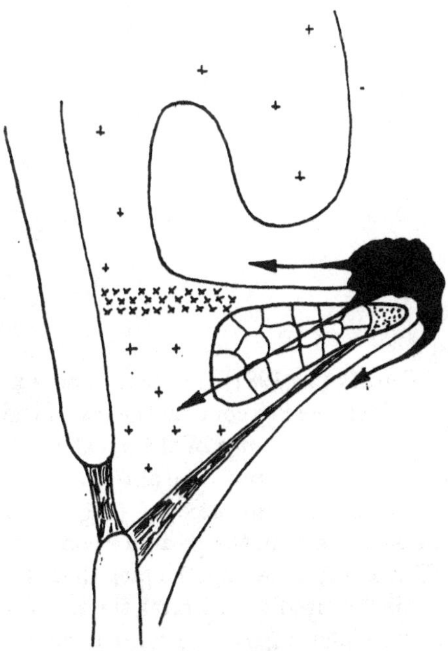

Fig. 34. Pathways of glottic cancer

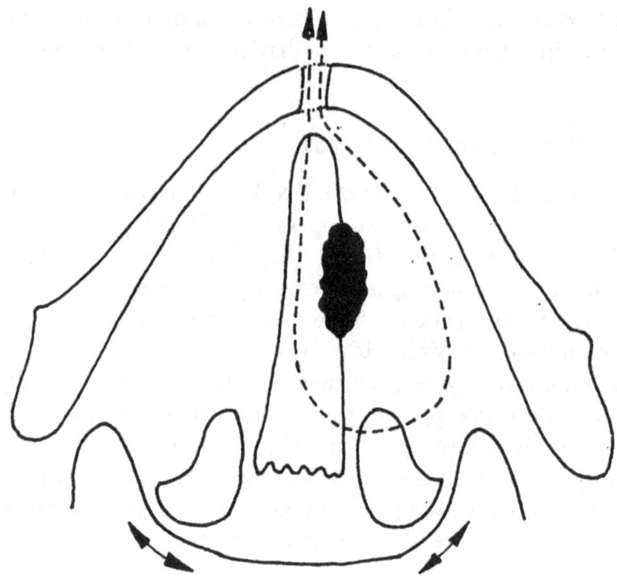

Fig. 35a. Scheme of extralaryngeal chordectomy

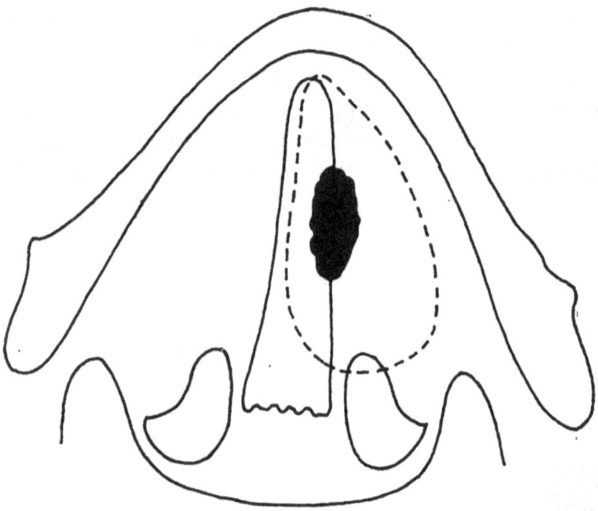

Fig. 35b. Scheme of endolaryngeal laser chordectomy

T_1 vocal cord tumours is not clearly defined yet BURIAN'S (1981) 18 operations, experience of JAKÓ et al. (1976) as well as our 112 operations seem to confirm the use of the laser. This is especially valid for T_1 tumours sitting on the free edge of the vocal cord, located in its middle third (Fig. 35c, d). Should the tumour infiltrate the anterior commissure, the anterior third of the contralateral vocal cord is also removed (Fig. 36b). In case of tumours located at the junction of the three cords or in the posterior commissure the laser chordectomy is not applied by us. This is explained by the fact that the T_{1b} tumour located in the anterior commissure relatively rapidly infiltrates the preepiglottic area (Fig. 34). The latter cannot be reached by endolaryngeal surgery. In tumours of the posterior commissure – also due to the direction of tumour infiltration – chordectomy

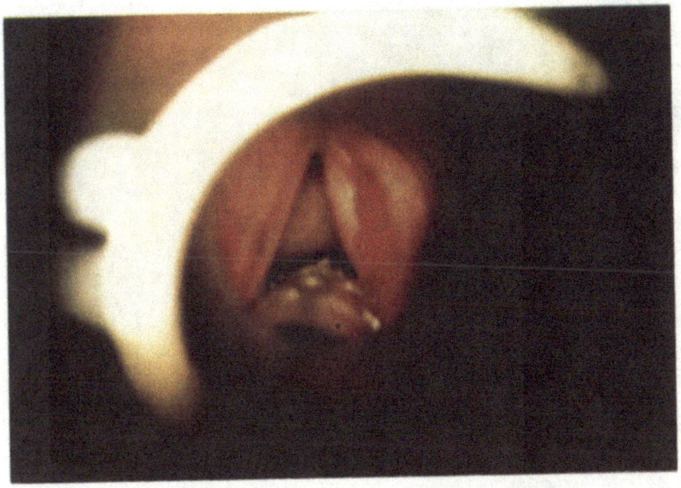

Fig. 35c. Vocal cord tumour T_{1a} before laser surgery

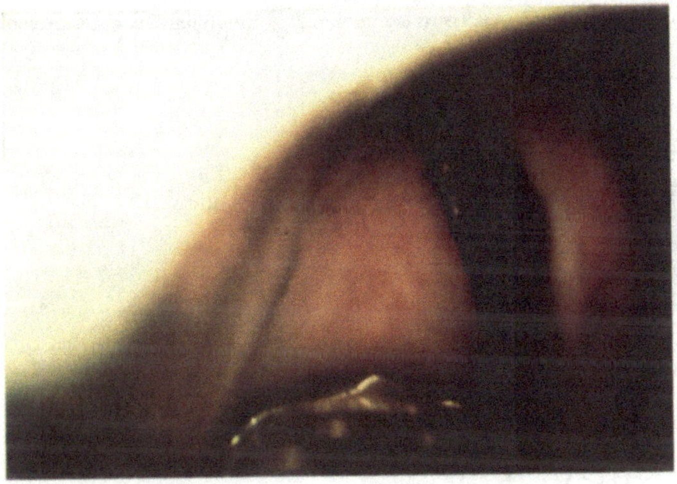

Fig. 35d. Vocal cord tumour T_{1a} after laser surgery

is not sufficent. It does not mean that BURIAN's (1981) procedure combined with radiotherapy or JAKÓ's (1979) radical attitude are not worth considering (Figs. 36b, 37b). In our own practice endolaryngeal laser surgery for T_{1b} tumours and that of the posterior commissure is performed only if the patient refuses the extralaryngeal radical operation. In such cases – provided the patient's consent is obtained – postoperative irradiation is performed. In the opposite case the classical procedure is followed (Figs. 36a, 28a).

In T_2 vocal cord cancer the chordectomy is insufficient, in these cases extended chordectomy or hemilaryngectomy should be done (BURIAN et al. 1981). This type of surgery includes the removal of tumorously infiltrated tissues together with the adequate safety zone. The extent of resection therefore depends on the site and extension of the tumorous process. If the T_2 process is unilateral and infiltrates the vestibular fold the endolaryngeal extended laser chordectomy may be indicated. However, in case the T_2 tumour also infiltrates the anterior commissure, posterior commissure, epiglottis, Morgagni's ventricle or the subglottis, the ablasticity of endolaryngeal surgery is highly

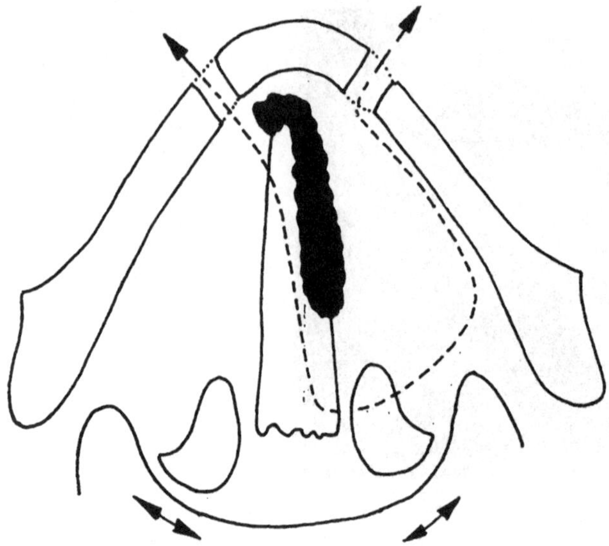

Fig. 36a. Scheme of conservative surgery of vocal cord carcinoma $T_{1,2}$ involving the anterior commissure

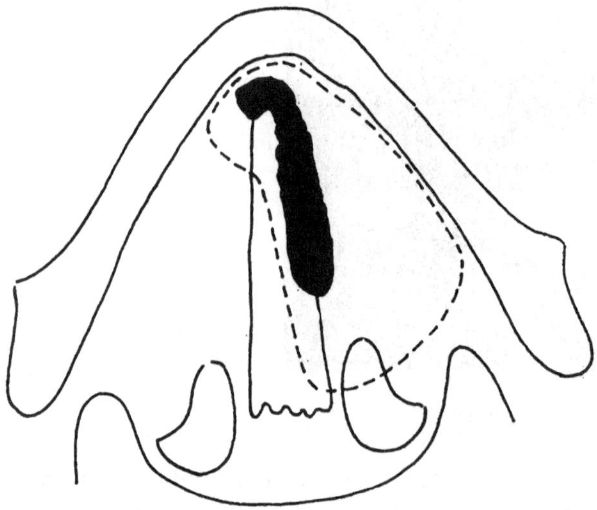

Fig. 36b. Scheme of laser surgery of vocal cord carcinoma $T_{1,2}$ involving the anterior commissure

questionable. In the latter case we perform endolaryngeal CO_2 laser surgery only if the patient refuses the extralaryngeal extended procedure. In each case following extended chordectomy postoperative irradiation is indicated. It is to be pointed out that several investigators regard the endolaryngeal laser operations of the T_2 vocal cord cancers as definitive. There is agreement, however, about the exclusively palliative purpose of the endolaryngeal laser surgery in $T_{3,4}$ tumours. It can be indicated only if the patient refuses radical surgery or it cannot be performed. In such cases the operation is aimed at temporarily ensuring the laryngeal lumen passage, i.e. prolonging tracheotomy. The radical extralaryngeal surgery of $T_{3,4}$ tumours can be performed by the handpiece of the laser instrument. The operative technique and the experiences are identical with

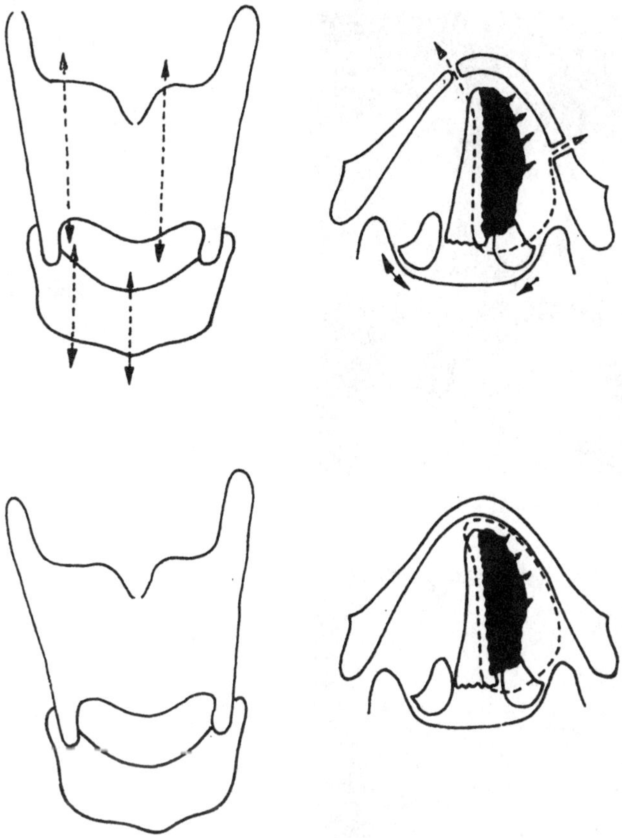

Fig. 37. Scheme of conservative surgery of vocal cord carcinoma $T_{1,2}$ involving the posterior commissure

those in case of extralaryngeal laser surgery of supraglottic tumours (Figs. 38a, b). For the endolaryngeal or extended chordectomy the lumen of the larynx is excellently explorable with laryngoscope. In the latter case the laryngoscope is not inserted too deeply and, if needed, the tube is set in another position.

The literature data unequivocally establish that the operative field is endolaryngeally perfectly explorable, the hit safety is 100%, the technique is "no-touch". The incision depth of the continuous laser beam of 30 to 40 W energy can be regulated. The operative field is bloodless and sterile. Suction of the steam should be ensured accordingly. Postoperative edema is almost entirely absent, no tracheotomy should be performed, the frame of the larynx need not be disrupted. The wound healing is adequate and rapid such as the epithelization of the operative field. Since there is no considerable scar formation, the functional result following laser chordectomy is good, the quality of voice is hardly changed. The intervention requires about 15 to 25 minutes, the "poor risk" patients can also be operated on. Hospitalization is about 2 to 3 days, which is financially highly beneficial to the health service and the patients have to wait less. (In case of our 112 patients this means, during 4 years, more than 700 days gained compared to the 21 nursing days following conventional chordectomy.)

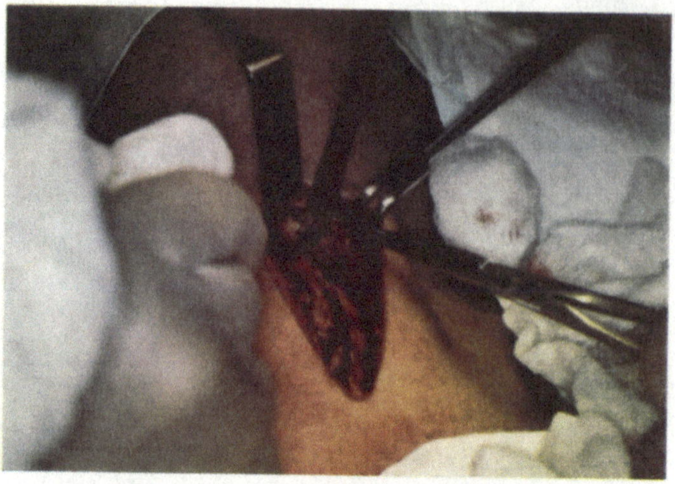

Fig. 38a. Median incision in laser laryngectomy

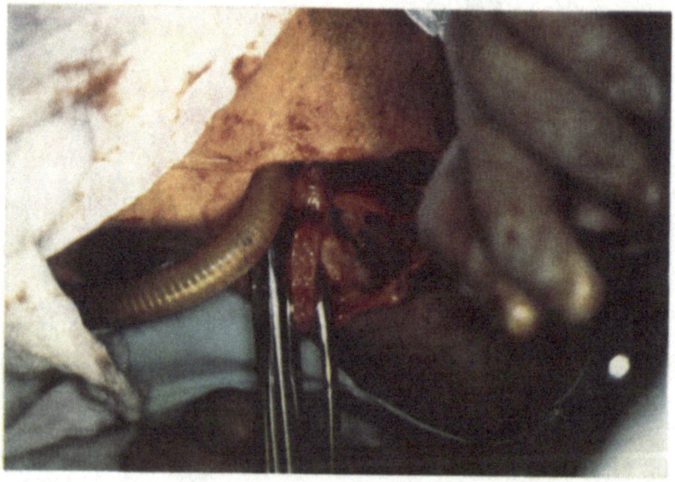

Fig. 38b. Laser laryngectomy; lifting of the larynx and dissection of the posterior wall

Of our 112 patients with T_1 vocal cord cancer undergone laser surgery, the specimen taken from the operative site at the end of surgery proved histologically positive in 12 cases. These patients received postoperative irradiation of 65 to 68 Gy/6 weeks. Out of them 11 patients are tumour-free after 3 years, in 1 patient recurrence of the primary tumour developed. In 100 patients with negative histology 4 local recurrences developed, in 2 of them the tumour persisted even after postoperative irradiation. In all relapsing patients laryngectomy was performed.

Due to T_2 glottic tumour 6 endolaryngeal operations were performed with laser. All the 6 patients received postoperative irradiation of 65 to 68 Gy/6 weeks. Four of them became tumour-free over 3 years, 2 developed local recurrence in 1 year. The latter refused laryngectomy and died within 2 years.

Due to T_3 glottic tumour 4 laser laryngectomies were performed. The 4 patients are locally tumour-free after 3 years.

The laser treatment of the ligamentary located T_{1a} carcinomas is an evidently successful new therapeutic form. Our experience – like that of others – suggests that the laser treatment of T_{1a} vocal cord carcinomas of the localizations described can bring about at least identical result with those after conventional methods. This can be stated also considering that the 3- or 5-year survival, oncologically regarded as correct, could be evaluated only in a limited number of patients.

Based on his 10-year experience JAKÓ establishes that the endolaryngeal laser surgery also in T_2 vocal cord tumours can be accepted as an oncologically equivalent or superior therapeutic alternative. In his opinion, the residual tumour after irradiation can be successfully treated by laser, furthermore, laser can be used for the management of recurrences as well.

4.12.10.3. Subglottic tumours

Our therapeutic principles in case of subglottic laryngeal tumours are as follows:

T_{is}, T_{1a}, T_{1b}	partial subglottic resection (rare) and postoperative irradiation
T_2, T_3	laryngectomy and postoperative irradiation
T_4	extended laryngectomy, with hypopharyngeal, tracheal, skin resection and postoperative irradiation in inoperable case: palliative irradiation and/or cytostatic treatment
N_1, N_2	radical neck dissection in monoblock
N_3	cytostatic treatment

The situation is similar in the subglottic laryngeal tumours as in the epiglottic ones. If histology is positive for the tumour there is a danger of the infiltration of the cartilage, too. Accordingly, only those tumours in the T_{is} group can undergo endolaryngeal laser surgery which can be completely visualized through laryngoscope, then removed by laser. Tumours not meeting these criteria can be safely managed only extralaryngeally, by laryngofission. We performed endolaryngeal laser surgery of T_{is} subglottic cancer in 2 cases. Both were localized under the anterior third of the vocal cord. With the usual exploration and operation techniques chordectomy was applied in a way that the tumour located a few mm-s beneath the vocal cord and the surrounding, apparently normal mucosa were vaporized. The mucosa of the anterior commissure was saved. No tracheotomy was performed. The wound healing was rapid, no significant adhesion developed. Subsequently, irradiation with a total tumour dose was given. The patients are tumour-free over 2 years.

In case of $T_{1a,b}$ subglottic tumours it is feasible to perform partial resection already from laryngofission. This ensures good exploration, easy handling of the handpiece and the radical extirpation of the tumour. Postoperative irradiation is indicated.

In case of $T_{2,3,4}$ subglottic tumours, too, extralaryngeal operations are to be performed. The procedure and experience when using the laser handpiece are also identical with those after supraglottic extralaryngeal surgery.

4.12.10.4. Palliative laryngosurgery

Radical laryngeal operations are frequently impossible to perform for various reasons (e.g., the patient's consent is lacking, oncological or anesthesiological contraindications, etc.). In these cases palliation with laser–though duration and rate of survival are unaffected - may temporarily ensure free upper respiratory tract, consequently no tracheotomy is needed. This indication is accepted by the majority of investigators. The technical execution of lumen-ensuring surgery is evidently determined by the site and extent of the constrictive tumour.

4.12.11. Stenoses of the upper respiratory tract

4.12.11.1. Laryngeal stenoses

A relatively rare and late complication developing probably as a consequence of inflammation or injury following the partial laryngeal resection due to laryngeal carcinomas is the synechia. Since 1964 in our 31 patients of 974 who had undergone laryngeal surgery we observed marked scarring causing synechia or laryngeal stenosis. In addition to this, 7 patients were transferred to us from other departments due to postoperative synechia. The cases of recurrent paraplegia are not included in this group. These synechiae were treated by extralaryngeal surgery up to the end of 1980. Since then, we have diagnosed 9 synechiae and operated on endolaryngeally with the CO_2 laser (Bánhidy et al. 1982). The use of the CO_2 laser in these cases is indicated by the significantly smaller scar formation compared with the conventional manipulations, thus the success of the laser synechiolysis could be assumed. The larynx is explored by the same method described previously. Then, synechiolysis is performed with 30 W of laser energy, with constant visual control (Fig. 39a, b). The scar was removed to the cartilage, and the patient was extubated. The operations lasted for 10 to 15 minutes and proved to be technically very simple. In the direct postoperative period the patient was able to communicate, no special therapy was applied. Although minimal scar formation could be observed on the operative field, respiration of the patients became satisfactory.

Miehlke and Vollrath (1980) also achieved favourable results by lasing the glottic and subglottic synechia and "sail-like" stenoses. For the definitive removal of larger, mainly subglottic stenoses, however, the laser is not considered suitable (because of the frequent recurrences). We have somewhat different opinion and experience since we managed by laser large subglottic stenoses in 2 cases. In one of the patients the intervention brought about definitive accomplishment. In the other patient repeated laser surgery in 2 sessions became necessary, in the course of which sylastic *T*-tube was inserted in the trachea.

Burian et al. (1981) reports on favourable results principally in childhood synechiolyses. The technically simple operations must be favourably evaluated since none of the other procedures lead to similar accomplishments. In childhood synechiolyses the absence of postoperative edema, the avoidance of tracheotomy, thus the prevention of late laryngeal deformities are of special significance.

In case of the endolaryngeal lasing of bilateral recurrent paraplegias, besides chordectomy, the arytenoid cartilage must be exarticulated – not vaporized – since this is the only solution for preventing the development of large bullous edema. In our clinic the traditional procedure is Réthi's glottic dilation operation. Developing Réthi's I. operation we perform arytenoidectomy and removal of the scarry vocal cord muscles. This is in most cases completed with Réthi's II. operation which means the transection of the posterior chondrous laryngeal wall and of the first or second tracheal cartilages, then traction of the halved larynx and retention in the new position. When performing

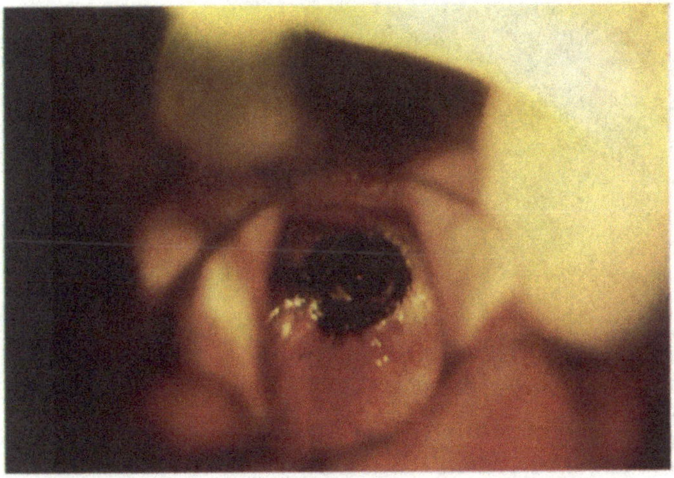

Fig. 39a. Synechiolysis with laser – first phase of surgery

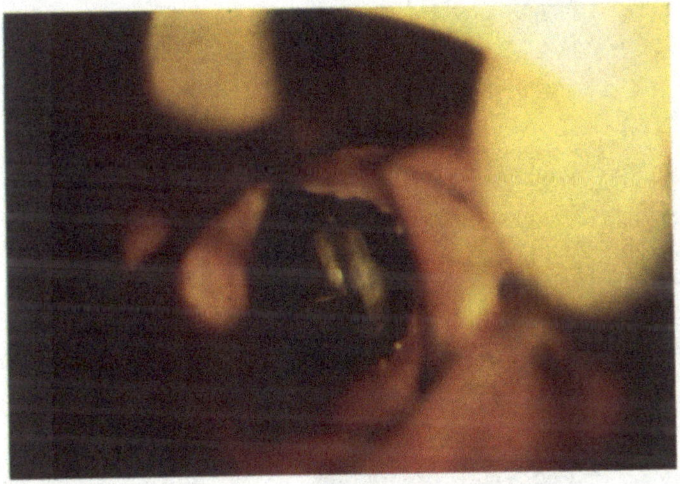

Fig. 39b. Synechiolysis with laser – last phase of surgery; the alfol covered tube inserted through the tracheostoma is visible

Réthi's operation I endolaryngeally by laser, the exarticulation and removal of the arytenoid cartilage may cause technical difficulty. It is advisable to perform chordectomy at first, thus the arytenoid cartilage can be approached on a bloodless operative field (Fig. 40a, b, c). Since the postoperative edema is minimal, tracheotomy need not be performed. If Réthi's operations I–II are performed in one session the extralaryngeal way must be chosen. The laryngofission is performed by the laser handpiece, then the assistant pulls the two halves of the larynx to lateral direction. Thus the laryngeal lumen is explored and Réthi's I–II operation is easily performed with the handpiece of the laser. Prior to implanting the glottic dilatator, it is feasible to place a Mikulicz-pad into the laryngeal lumen. Following Réthi's I–II glottic dilatation laser surgery the wound healing was adequate, no inflammation was observed.

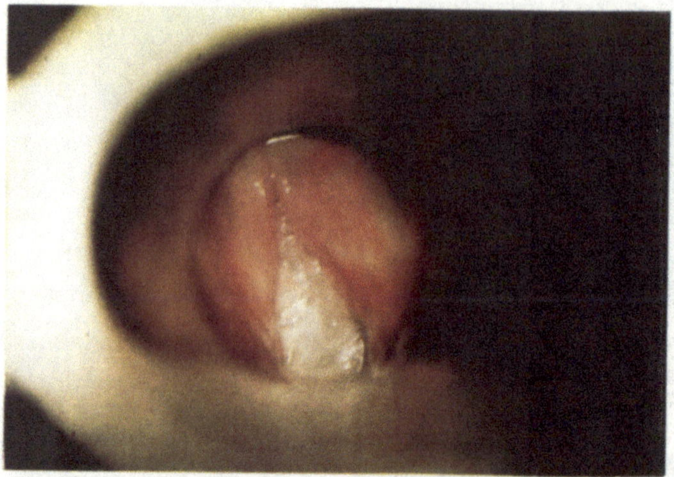

Fig. 40a. Paraplegia of both recurrent laryngeal nerves – intubation

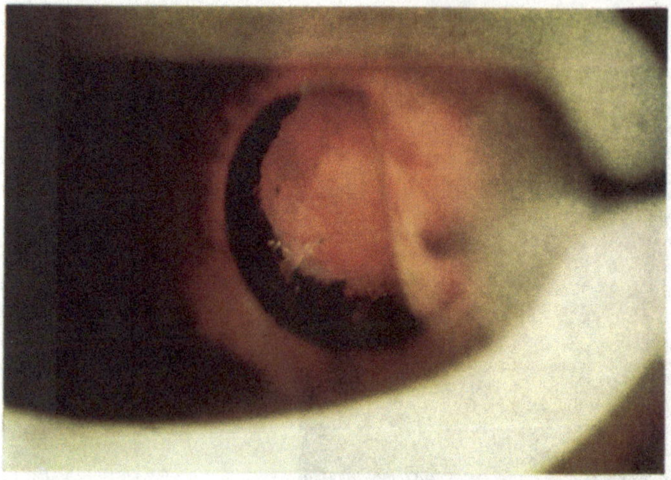

Fig. 40b. Paraplegia of both recurrent laryngeal nerves – removal of one vocal cord by laser

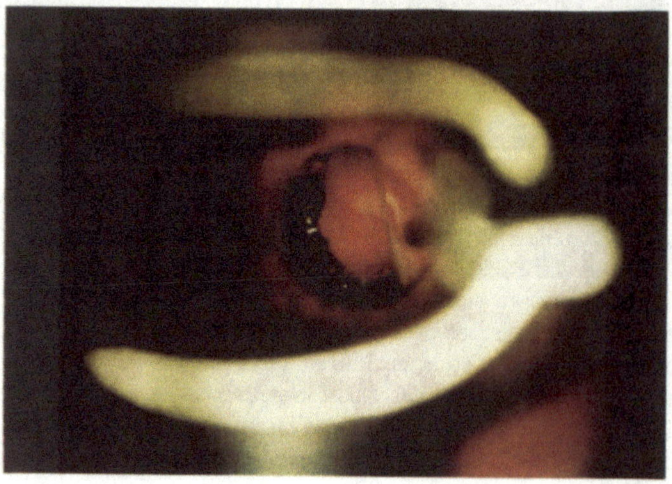

Fig. 40c. Paraplegia of both recurrent laryngeal nerves – condition after arytenoidectomy

4.12.11.2. Tracheal stenoses

Stenoses of the upper trachea can be divided into 2 major groups: stenoses caused by exterior or interior compression that may result from a great variety of diseases. Among them only those can be operated on endotracheally with the CO_2 laser which can be explored by Kleinsasser-or Weerda-laryngoscope or are accessible by the laser beam and in case the surgery is oncologically not contraindicated.

These are the benign lesions of the uppermost part of the trachea. In our opinion, of the obstructing stenotizing processes, only the benign tumours, the postintubation granulomas can be treated by the CO_2 laser. The mode of surgery is identical with that applied for laryngeal stenoses.

In our department 3 endotracheal CO_2 laser operations have been performed due to benign tumour and 3 due to intubation granulomas. Our experience is as favourable as in the endolaryngeal synechiolyses by the CO_2 laser.

The obstructive malignant tumours of the upper trachea must be, in our opinion, subject to conventional surgical interventions, the laser operation can be only of palliative character. In case of tracheomalacia or exterior compressive stenosis we perform surgery or apply sylastic endoprosthesis.

4.13. Cancer of the hypopharynx

The hypopharyngeal cancer accounts for 0.6 to 3% of all malignancies. More than 90% of the cases is squamous cell carcinoma. Its very poor prognosis can be explained by the lack of symptoms, late diagnosis, resistance to irradiaton and formation of metastases also to the mediastinum.

Our therapeutic principles followed in hypopharyngeal tumours are listed below:

T_{is}, T_1 radiotherapy or hypopharyngeal resection

T_2 radiotherapy or
in case of tumours of the sinus pyriformis and posterior wall: hypopharyngeal resection in case of sinus pyriformis, posterior wall and retrocricoideal tumours: hypopharyngeal resection with laryngectomy

T_3 hypopharyngeal resection with laryngectomy (rarely hypopharyngeal extirpation and plastic reconstruction) and postoperative irradiation

T_4 removal of the larynx and hypopharynx and reconstruction of the pharynx (PM flap) and postoperative irradiation
in inoperable cases: tracheotomy, palliative irradiation and/or cytostatic treatment

N_1N_2 radical neck dissection in monoblock

N_3 palliative irradiation and/or administration of cytostatics

In the surgical treatment of all hypopharyngeal cancers only the handpiece of the laser can be used. Not only the endoscopic exploration but the correct management of the operative field are extremely difficult.

In case of malignoma the line of resection must be beyond the safety zone, it is not enough to remove the lesion superficially. Since the wall of the hypopharynx has only two layers, in view of the deep infiltration, the hypopharyngeal wall must also be resected. This cannot be done by endoscope. Reconstruction of the luminal continuity is also impossible.

The laser operation of hypopharyngeal tumours can be performed only by using the handpiece. The type of resection and reconstruction depends on the site and extent of the tumour. As to the technical problems and experience we refer to the extralaryngeal surgery of the laryngeal tumours. Considering that the entrance of the hypopharynx-oesophagus can be reconstructed mostly by myocutaneous flap, lacking experience, we assume that the wound healing is similar to that described in connection with the reconstruction of the skin and oral cavity.

4.14. Laser surgery of the cervical structures

4.14.1. Tracheotomy

In the last decades the indication of tracheotomy has changed. The role of acute tracheotomy has been virtually taken over by the intubation of the patients. In those cases, however, when the airways cannot be steadily kept open otherwise (e.g., due to tumorous, scarry, paralytic stenosis) and the patient suffocates, tracheotomy is performed immediately. The use of laser is particularly advantageous in transtumoral tracheotomy. This is most frequently performed, in case of inoperable thyroid cancer (Fig. 41a, b, c, d). Tracheotomy performed through the advanced thyroid carcinoma is especially difficult because the tumour is generally richly vascularized, the hemostasis is difficult, the cervical structures like the common and internal carotid artery, internal jugular vein, vagus nerve, recurrent laryngeal nerve, the wall of the hypopharynx are dislocated, thus the trachea is hardly accessible and the hazard of accessory injuries is great. Among the advantages of the laser those are taken use of in the tracheotomy by advanced thyroid carcinomas like e.g. that it immediately coagulates the blood vessels to 0.5 mm, thus the bleeding is minimal, the operative field is easy to explore, the structures are easy to recognize, manage or save. The following procedure of laser tracheotomy is performed in our clinic (KÁSLER et al. 1982). Following anesthesia the anesthesiologist intubates the patient, by using Rüsch-tube. It is firm enough to support the tracheal wall and to promote the intraoperative orientation. Subsequently, we cut through the

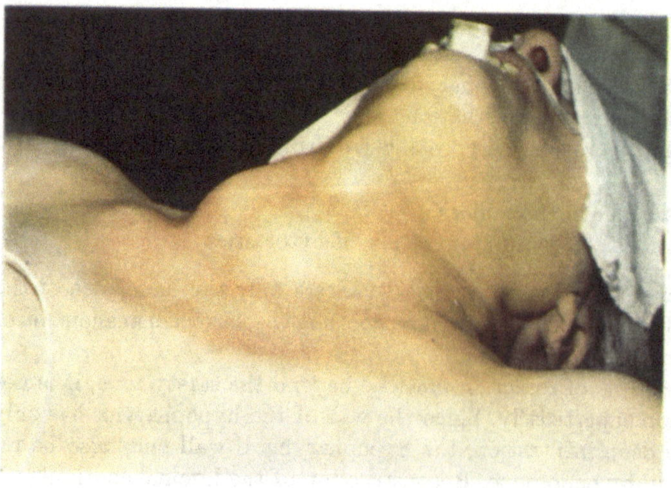

Fig. 41a. Malignant goiter causing tracheal compression

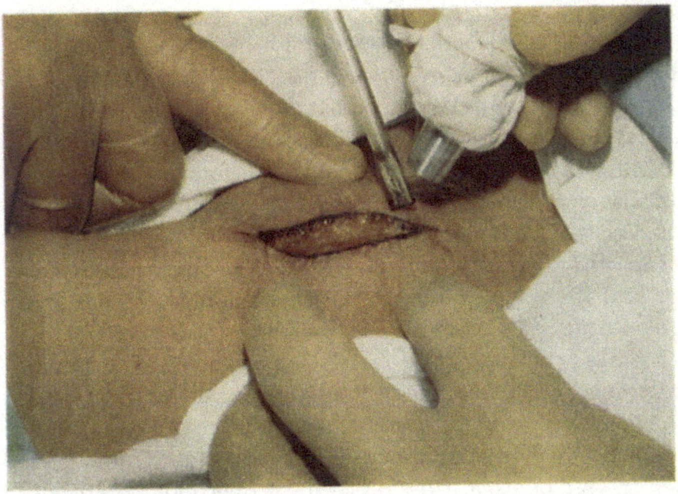

Fig. 41b. Skin incision

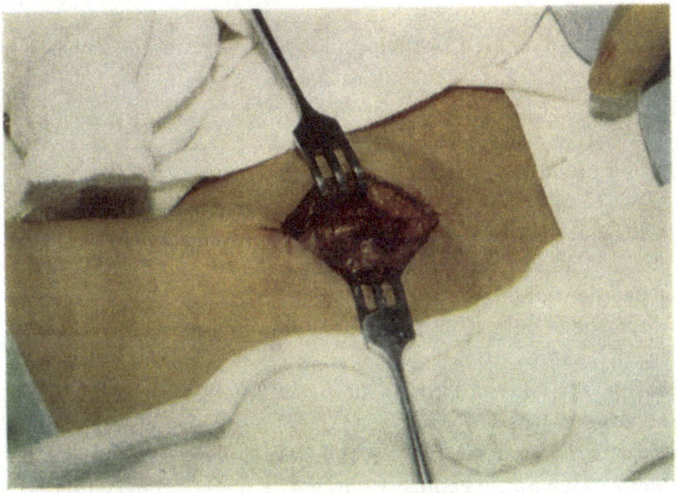

Fig. 41c. Dissection of the tumour, search for the trachea

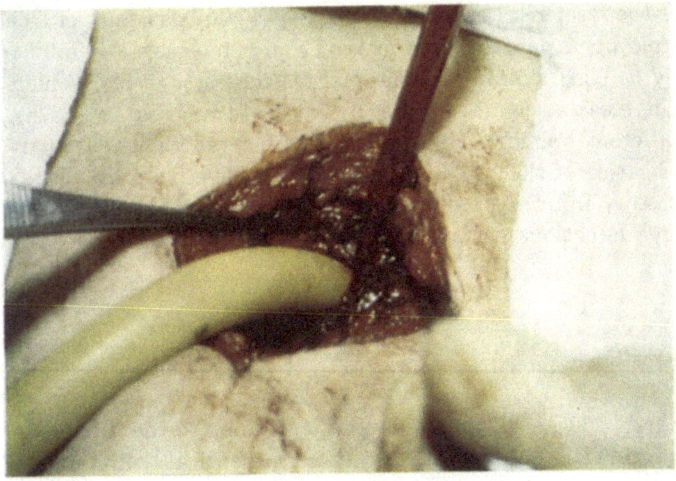

Fig. 41d. Transtubation of the patient

skin by the laser handpiece and, with the continuous traction of the wound edges, proceed towards the trachea. The wound surface incised by the laser is almost entirely dry. When reaching the tracheal wall the administration of narcotics is discontinued, by satisfactory spontaneous respiration the patient is extubated and the tracheal wall is transected only afterwards. This is because the laser beam may perforate the tube and the gas narcotics may explode. The concentration of the oxygen at spontaneous breathing is only about 20%, thus the danger of explosion is not threatening.

For transection of the tracheal wall there are only a few seconds at our disposal since the anesthesia is almost over and the oxygenization of the patient must be ensured. Surgery is completed by implantation of a cannula and packing of the wound.

By this procedure we have operated on 5 patients so far. The operations lasted 20 minutes on the average, they were simple and were not associated with any accessory injuries. In addition to that, the operation was bloodless, the cervical structures were easy to identify, postoperative local edema and necrosis were not encountered.

The tracheotomy performed in case of stenotizing processes is operation technically identical with that for struma maligna but the hazard of accessory injuries is incomparably smaller, the loss of blood is minimal.

The laser tracheotomy may be of great significance under warlike circumstances or in case of infected cervical wounds.

4.14.2. Surgery of the thyroid gland

There may be various indications of these operations. Without going into detail, the thyroid hyperfunction, compression following tissue enlargement of any type and the tumorous degeneration must be mentioned.

The major types of surgery are the enucleation, the different wedge-resections, lobectomy and the total thyroid extirpation.

The greatest danger of these operations is caused by the fact that the thyroid gland is located in the vicinity of vital organs (see tracheotomy). The enlarged glandular substance may dislocate these structures therefore their recognition is often very difficult. The glandular substance is rich in blood and bleeding occurring at resection may further hinder the intraoperation orientation.

The greatest advantage of the laser resection is the hemostasis. Christensen (1976) used the CO_2 laser in 7 thyroid operations for skin incision and hemostasis at the line of resection. Intraoperatively he used mainly conventional instruments. In his opinion the use of the laser does not mean a significant benefit. Glantz and Korn (1976), however, are of completely different opinion. The extirpated tissue was highly vascularized, they used laser by the ligature of the major vessels. The operative field was bloodless, well-explorable, no accessory injuries were seen, the postoperative period was uneventful. The 3 thyroid wedge resections performed in our clinic seem to support the latter opinion and experience.

4.14.3. Radical neck dissection

The common feature of the head and neck tumours is that, according to the rule of involvement of satellites, they form their regional metastases in the cervical lymph nodes. The oncologically accepted surgery of the cervical metastases is the radical neck dissection (RND). This means the complete removal of all cervical lymph nodes; on the relevant side above the deep cervical fascia only the carotid artery system, the vagus nerve and the hypoglossal nerve are saved. The operation is classified into medium-large category, the preservation of the structures requires fastidious preparation. Since the laser is hardly suitable for fine preparation, only a few surgeons (FRIEDMAN 1976, ARANOFF 1976) performed this operation. Their experience corresponds to that obtained with the handpiece in the laser surgery of soft tissues.

4.14.4. Parotid tumours

The laser surgery of these tumours differs from the others in respect that, close to the facial nerve the preparation must be continued by conventional instruments, to prevent the thermal damage of the nerve and the secondary facial paraplegia. In case the facial nerve is tumorously infiltrated or its histological character justifies its removal, the nerve must be resected and reconstructed. In such a case it must be considered how the laser-cut surface influences the result of the nerve reconstruction. The same relates to the laser removal of head and neck tumours of nerve origin (e.g., transseptal hypophysectomy).

5. The Low-energy Laser in the Otorhinolaryngology

5.1. Laser therapy of chronic tonsillitis

The chronic tonsillitis is most often caused by the streptococcal beta-hemolytic strains. In the compensated stage only the tonsil shows inflammatory changes while the prolonged inflammation and its progression leads to the decompensation of the process and to the chronic inflammation of distant organs (rheuma, nephritis, polyarthritis). The therapy of compensated tonsillitis is essential for preventing the development of the hardly curable, severe processes and consequences of the decompensation. The individual forms (antibiotics, tonsillectomy, etc.) of conservative treatment have both advantages and disadvantages, there is no fully beneficial treatment available. This fact gave the notion of examining the applicability of the CO_2 laser and determining its place among the other therapeutic procedures. First the effect of laser of 0.337 μm wavelength on the beta hemolytic, standard streptococcal strain was studied. It was found that the reproduction acivity of the standard strains decreased at the energy level of 5 mW/cm^2. Similarly, the hemolytic and hyaluronidase activity also diminished.

When increasing the energy further, in the range of 5 to 10 mW/cm^2, by an exposition time of 15 minutes the viability of the bacteria ceased. In this range of energy and by this exposition time no morphological changes occurred on the tissues irradiated.

After selecting the most successfully applicable type of laser, determining the dose of irradiation, performing the morphological and biochemical studies the method was used in clinical practice in 305 cases.

Favourable experience could be gained:

1. The laser treatment killed the streptococcal beta-hemolytic strains.
2. The tonsillitis eliminated.
3. The tonsil and adjacent tissues did not get damaged, their tissue structure regenerated soon.
4. The treatment is painless.
5. It can be performed on outpatient basis, too.

In order to apply this method also in unfavourable topographic situation a fiberoscopic, photoconductive system was developed, ensuring access to the tonsil in any variety of cases. The method is regarded as part of the complex therapy and successful for compensated chronic tonsillitis. The limitations of the laser treatment in case of decompensated inflammations is, however, emphasized.

5.2. Laser therapy of the defects of the external ear

It has become evident from many investigations that the low-energy laser increases the fibroblast activity, the phagocytosis, the collagen synthesis and stimulates the circulation of the regenerating tissues. This gave the idea of treating by laser the injuries induced on the eardrum of guinea pigs of 400 to 500 g body weight. The animals were divided into 2 groups. In the first group triangular defects of equal size were formed on both eardrums of the animals. In the individuals of the other group the bilateral perforation was closed by myringoplastics with fascia and, to support the transplant, gelfoam was placed into the tympanic cavity. After denudation of the perforative wound edge the fascia was located between the gelfoam and the eardrum. In the first group the edge of the perforation was unilaterally lasered for 5 minutes every second day, the other side was the control. The same procedure took place in the other group. The wavelength of the He-Ne laser was 632.8 μm, the power density 1.3 mW, the transection of the laser beam 1 mm², respectively. Irradiation was performed through operation microscope by a speculum system. Following irradiation the eardrum of decapitated animals was histologically examined. Epithelization proved considerably faster on the lased edge of the defect than on the control side. Duration of the complete closure varied with the size of defect and the number of treatments. In the control group II the fascial grafts adhered on the lasered side about twice as frequently as on the other (of 11 the ratio was 9:5). In addition, the duration of the complete incorporation was shorter. The histological findings did not reveal laser-specific changes.

Researches in 81 cases applied the He-Ne laser of 20 to 25 mW power output and 10 to 15 mW/cm² power density for stimulating the incorporation of tympanic grafts. The duration of irradiation was 5 minutes. Its success was evaluated on the basis of incidence of homograft incorporation, thermometric results, speed of recovery as well as the cytological cytochemical and bacteriological examination of the wound discharge. The treatment seems to activate the intracellular enzyme system, to increase the number of cells and the enzyme activity of the developing cells. Thus, the new microcirculation builds up rapidly, the graft incorporates quickly and with high frequency.

In experiments on dogs and rats Escudero et al. (1979) determined the type of laser, energy, exposition time and cross sections of beam of rays to be used in case of tympanoplastics.

Based on clinical and histological studies they compared the results obtained by optimal laser parameters to those after the use of electrocauter. In view of their favourable experience the laser was introduced in the human tympanoplastics. If the defect of the tympanic membrane was small, the operative field was accessible through the external auditory passage, in case of large defects the classical postauricular approach described by Portmann was used. In the latter case numerous venous bleedings can be expected, causing the following difficulties to the surgeon:

1. Bleedings encumber the visibility of the operative field and the performance of surgery.
2. Following the implantation of the temporal fascia the developing hematoma dislocates the graft and may even cause extrusion.

The conventional management of bleedings by electrocauter is difficult and time-consuming. Besides, the electrocauter not only coagulates the vessels but damages the surrounding soft tissues as well.

Following excision of the fascial graft it should be set in correct position on the recipient area, and to avoid dislocation it should be embedded in absorptive gelatin.

The argon laser beam of 500 to 1000 mW and 100 μm in diameter was used for hemostasis in 7 human tympanoplastics. The exposition time was 0.2 sec. Under operation microscope, the vessels were coagulated by laser from postauricular approach. The hemostasis was successful. The insignificant thermal damage of the adjacent tissues was confirmed also by the rapid healing of patients, as it was seen in animal experiments. After the implantation of the temporal fasica, the tympanic area was treated by laser beam of 560 mW energy and 0.2 to 0.5 sec exposition time. The incidental adhesions, tissue damage and microvascularization were controlled. The control examinations proved the adequate position and incorporation of the neotympanum. Extrusion was not encountered, the internal ear did not get damaged. The audiometric examinations confirmed proper function.

Of another 7 tympanoplastics in 6 cases perfect incorporation of the temporal fascial graft was seen. Various types of laser were applied for the treatment of different diseases of the external and middle ear. The experiences are favourable.

5.3. Laser treatment of the otosclerosis

The well approved therapy of otospongiosis implying the fixation of the sole of the stapes through stapedectomy. In 1 to 2% of the surgically treated patients postoperative sensoneural impaired hearing develops. Among the numerous causes the insufficient operative technique, the direct acoustic damage of the organ of hearing, the postoperative serous labyrinthitis, the perilymphatic fistule, the oval window granuloma, the coexistent cochlear otospongiosis, etc. are to be mentioned. The partial stapedectomy and the stapedectomy reduce the operative traumatization and the hazard of damaging the internal ear structures. The great advantage of the laser stapedectomy over the manual manipulation is the no-touch procedure, the minimal operative traumatization, the bloodless operative field and good visibility. The severe danger of its application is the thermal damage of the internal ear structures.

To clarify this question Coker et al. (1985) conducted animal experiments. Under ketamine anesthesia, the vestibulum of cats was explored by diamond drill, under the oval window. Then fenestration was performed by the CO_2 laser. The animals were divided in 2 groups. In the first group the power output was 0.47 to 3.05 W, the time of exposition 0.5 sec. These values were 0.51 to 3.05 W and 0.2 sec in the second group, respectively. The focal point of the laser beam was 150 μm diameter. The changes of temperature in the vestibulum were separately registered in case of perforative and non-perforative laser doses. Out of 46 laser impulses 12 penetrated the sole of the stapes. Fenestration took place by 1.69 W, the thermal damage was insignificant. By 2.3 W the perilymph was boiling, above 3.05 W rapid vaporization started and tissue defect formed towards the vestibulum. Therefore, the power applied must not exceed 3.05 W. In case of 1.0 W the warming of the sole of the stapes is merely 1.1°C, no penetration occurs, consequently, this low level of power is unsuitable for stapedectomy. It is proved by experiments that the power output of 2.2 W, by an exposition time of 0.2 sec consequently causes penetration in a way that the perilymph does not boil and the thermal change of the vestibulum is only 1.1°C. The correlation between the laser power, exposition time, the short interval between laser impulses and the increase of temperature was found evident.

In guinea pigs and cats the change of chochlear activity during argon and Ne-YAG laser stapedectomy and for 2 months afterwards was measured. No significant difference was detected between the classical and laser procedures.

The promontorium of 10 guinea pigs was irradiated by argon laser of 0.6 to 2.2 W, with an exposition time of 0.5 sec. At the same time, the brain stem potential evoked by the bone conduction as well as the cochlear temperature were registered.

While the former experimental results were influenced by the perilymphatic fistula and operative trauma induced by the measuring instruments, the latter ones registered the effect of laser on the organ of Corti and the laser load capacity of the internal ear. It means that not only the higher temperature may cause the damage of the internal ear but in the course of irradiation the gas developing under the attained bone evokes rapid change of pressure in the endocochlear fluid. Thus the thermal increase is not a direct but an indirect damaging factor. It was supported by the fact that no morphological changes could be observed following laser treatment of the stria vascularis. Another series of investigations led to controversial conclusions. The laser effect was photodocumented through a microscope of 40x-3 magnification. The animals were sacrificed between 5 hours to 3 days or 3 to 5 weeks, the stria vascularis was isolated and histologically studied. Significant vascular changes were found, but they were reversible under 100 mW power and 1 sec exposition time or they were irreversible on the stria vascularis without damaging the organ of Corti. In case of higher values impaired hearing must be reckoned with.

PERKINS (1980) who was the first to apply argon laser for stapedectomy, – the diameter of the beam was 50 to 100 μm, exposition time 100 msec, the power 0.4 to 0.7 W – reported on excellent results in 11 treated patients.

McGEE (1983) performed 100 stapedectomies with argon laser of 1.5 W power output and 1.0 sec exposition time. After 6 months the bone conduction was identical or better than prior to surgery. After 1 year, however, there was no significant difference compared to the bone conduction of the 139 patients undergone conservative surgery. The favourable results of human stapedectomies were not confirmed by animal (e.g. cat) experiments. This is explained by the difference in the anatomic structure, inorganic substance and pigment content of the sole of stapes of man and cat.

Other investigators found cochlear lesion by a power higher than 0.8 W when applying the CO_2 laser of 1 to 25 mm in diameter, 0.4 to 1.6 W power and 0.5 sec exposition time. The extent of the lesion increased proportionally with the energy. In other studies the CO_2 laser of 400 μm in diameter and 15 msec exposition time was used for treating the middle and internal ear of monkeys and cadavers. By the higher range of energy and exposition time the stria vascularis becomes atrophic and the pilus cells of the Corti organ get destructed. In conclusion it is established that the CO_2 laser can be applied only by strict parameters of controlled power, output, energy, time of exposition, focal length and cross-section of beam.

Certain researchers recommend the use of the CO_2 laser of 2 to 4 W power and 0.05 sec exposition time for performing stapedectomy of 0.3 mm (based on cat experiments).

Theoretical considerations (parameter-dependent CO_2 laser effect on fluids and bones) and animal experiments suggest that the CO_2 laser of 0.5 to 3.0 W power, 150 μm diameter and 0.2 sec or shorter exposition time is suitable for performing stapedectomy, with negligible operative traumatization and thermal increase in the vestibulum.

6. References

Alcalay, A., Abastado, M., Dutron, C., Rosencher, N., Reyt, E., Junien-Lavillauroy, C.: La jet - ventilation pré - glottique dans la microchirurgie au laser. A propos de 100 cas: J. Franc. ORL. **33**, 196 (1984)

Albegger, K., Küttner, J.: Zum Problem der laserinduzierten Entflammung bei der endolaryngealen Microchirurgie aus gutachtlicher Sicht. Zentralbl. **130**, 5540 (1984)

Allgöver, M., Matter, P., Perren, S. M., Ruedi, T.: The dynamic compression plate. Springer-Verlag (1973)

Andrews, A. H.: Jewerly chain on cottonoids for CO_2 laser surgery. Ann. Otol. **88**, 827 (1979)

Andrews, A. H., Moss, H. W.: Experience with the carbon dioxide laser in the larynx. Ann. Otol. **83**, 462 (1974)

Andrews, A. H., Polanyi, T. G.: Microscopic and endoscopic surgery with the CO_2 laser. Boston-Bristol-London, John Wright PSG Inc. (1982)

Andrews, A. H., Polanyi, T. G., Grybauskas, V. T.: General techniques and clinical considerations in laryngologic laser surgery. Otolaryng. Clin. N. Amer. **16**, 793 (1983)

Annyas, A. A., Overbeek, J. J. M., et al.: CO_2 laser in malignant lesions of the larynx. Laryngoscope **94**, 836 (1984)

Albert, P. W.: The complications of CO_2 laser surgery in otolaryngology. Acta Otolaryngol. **91**, 375 (1981)

Apfelberg, D. B., Maser, M. R., Lash, H.: Review of usage of argon and carbon dioxide lasers for pediatric hemangiomas. Ann. Plast. Surg. **12**, 353 (1984)

Aronoff, B. L.: CO_2 laser in surgical oncology. Jerusalem Acad. Press. Jesus 133 (1978)

Aronoff, B. L.: CO_2 laser in surgical oncology. Internat. Adv. in Surg. Onc. **1**, 243 (1978)

Aronoff, B. L.: The carbon dioxide laser in head and neck and plastic surgery: Advantages and disadvantages. In: Goldman, L.: The biomedical laser. Springer, Berlin (1981)

Avellaneda, R., et al.: Estenosis laringeas postcirurgia oncologica. Tratamiento mediante Laser CO_2. Acta otorrinolaring esp. **35**, 437 (1984)

Babayan, R., Farthmann, E.: Laser und Wundheilung. Zbl. Chirurgie **102**, 1247 (1977)

Baló, J.: Kórbonctani és kórszövettani elváltozások a laser sugarak hatására. Orv. Hetil. **107**, 1016 (1966)

Bán, T.: A laserek müködésének fizikai alapjai. Orv. Hetil. **107**, 1009 (1966)

Bánhidy, F. G., Kásler, M., Boér, A., Rózsa, L.: Die Möglichkeit der Anwendung des chirurgischen Lasers in der HNO. Öster. HNO-Kongr. 162 (1985)

Bánhidy, F. G., Kásler, M., Zemplén, B., Pólus, K., Veszprémi, Z.: Über die CO_2-Laser-Therapie von Stenosen des Larynx und der Halstrachea. Wiss. Zeitschr. **33**, 243 (1984)

Belkahia, A.: Effets biologiques du faisceau laser en oto-laryngologie. Approche pour l'application médicale. Ann. Oto-Laryng. (Paris) **88**, 467 (1971)

Benn-Bassat, M., Kaplan, I., Shindel, Y., Edlan, A.: The CO_2 laser in surgery of the tongue. Jerusalem Acad. Press. Jesus 126 (1976)

Ben-Bassat, M., Kaplan, J, Shindel, Y., Edlan, A.: The CO_2 laser in surgery of the tongue. Brit. J. Plast. Surg. **31**, 155 (1978)

Benn-Bassat, M., Kaplan, I., Levy, R.: Treatment of hereditary haemorrhagic telangiectomia of the nasal mucosa with the carbon dioxide laser. Brit. J. Plast. Surg. **31**, 157 (1978)

BORGHESE, M. et al.: Impiego del laser a CO_2 del trattamento delle stenosi tracheali cicatrisiali. Otorinolar. (Torino) **34**, 433 (1984)

BOSCH, J., ZORITA, C., YOUNI, M.: El laser de CO_2 en microcirurgia laryngea. Acta otorrinolaring. esp. **34**, 233 (1983)

BRIGHTWELL, A. P.: A complication of the use of the laser in ENT surgery. J. Laryng. (London) **97**, 671 (1983)

BRONDBO, K., ALBERTI, P. W., CROWSON, M.: Adult recurrent multiple laryngeal papilloma: Laser management and socioeconomic effects. Acta Otolaryngol. **95**, 431 (1983)

BROPHY, J. W., SCULLY, P. A., STRATTON, C. J.: Argon laser use in papillomas of the larynx. Laryngoscope **92**, 1164 (1982)

BURGESS, G. E., LEJEUNE, F. E.: Endotracheal tube ignition during laser surgery of the larynx Arch. Otolaryngol. **105**, 561 (1979)

BURIAN, K.: CO_2-Laser in der Microchirurgie des Kehlkopfes. Laryng. Rhinol. **58**, 545 (1979)

BURIAN, K., HÖFLER, H.: Zur mikrochirurgischen Therapie von Stimmbandkarzinomen mit dem CO_2-Laser. Laryng. Rhinol. **58**, 551 (1979)

BURIAN, K., HÖFLER, H., LESSEL, M.: Endolaryngeale Mikrochirurgie mit dem CO_2-Laser. Zentralbl. **127**, 4210 (1981)

CAPELLÁ, G., ADEMÁ, J., GUIX, M.: Estudio experimental de las lesiibes oridzcudas por el rayo laser sobre la mucosa laringea de perro. Acta otorrhinolaring. esp. **34**, 98 (1983)

CARRUTH, J. A. S., MCKENZIE, A. L., WAINWRIGHT, A. C.: The carbon dioxide laser: safety aspets. J. Laryng. **94**, 411 (1980)

CARRUTH, J. A. S.: Resection of the tongue with the carbon dioxide laser. J. Laryng. **96**, 529 (1982)

CARRUTH, J. A. S.: The role of lasers in otolaryngology. World J. Surg. **7**, 719 (1983)

CARRUTH, J. A. S.: Laryngeal microsurgery with the carbon dioxide laser: Techniques and instrumentation. J. Laryng. **99**, 573 (1985)

CARRUTH, J. A. S.: Resection of the tongue with the carbon dioxide laser: 100 cases. J. Laryng. **99**, 887 (1985)

CASEY, K. R., FAIRMAX, W. R., SMITH, S. J. et al.: Intratracheal fire ignited by the ND-YAG laser during treatment of tracheal stenosis. Chest. **84**, 295 (1983)

CASTRO, D., STUART, A., BENVENUTI, D. et al.: A new method of dosimetry. – A study of comparative laser induced tissue damage. Ann. plast. Surg. **9**, 221 (1982)

CATALANO, G. B., ROSSI, M., SERRA, A. et al.: Laser o pinza ? A proposito di 50 casi di polipi e mixomi della laringe trattati con CO_2 lasermicrochirurgia. Otorhinolaring. ital. **33**, 15 (1983)

CERVELLERA, G., FORELLA, R.: Esperienze di microchirurgia laringea con laser CO_2. Otorinolaring. (Milano) **33**, 335 (1983)

CHRISTENSEN, J.: The Sharplan CO_2 laser in thoracic surgery. In KAPLAN, I.: Laser surgery. Academic Press. Jerusalem (1976)

COCHRANE, J. P., BEACON, Y. P., CREASEY, G. H.: Wound healing after laser surgery: an experimental study. Brit. J. Surg. **67**, 740 (1980)

COHEN, N. L.: A simple, inexpensive, disposable suction device for laser surgery. Otolaryng. Head Neck Surg. **89**, 451 (1981)

COKER, N. J., ATOR, G. A., JENKINS, H. A., NEBLETT, C. R., MORRIS, J. R.: Carbon dioxide laser stapedotomy. Arch. Otolaryngol. 601 (1985)

COTTON, R. T., TEWFIK, T. L.: Larynxstenose nach CO_2-laserbehandlung von subglottischen Hämangiomen. Ann. Otolaryng. (St. Louis) **94**, 494 (1985)

CROKETT, D. M., MCGILL, T. J. I., HEALY, G. B., FRIEDMAN, E. M.: Benign lesions of the nose? Oral cavity? and oropharynx in children: Excision by carbon dioxide laser. Ann. Otolaryng. (St. Louis) **94**, 489 (1985)

CROS, A. M., ESTEBEN, D., MEHSEN, M. et al.: La jet ventilation á haute fréquence: son interẽt au cours de la microchirurgie laryngée au laser CO_2 (á propos de 189 cas). Rev. Laryngoscope **104**, 209 (1983)

DAVIS, K. R., JAKÓ, G. J., HYAMS, V. J., SHAPSHAY, S. M.: The anatomic limitations of CO_2 laser cordectomy. Laryngoscope **92**, 980 (1982)

DAVIS, K. R., SIMPSON, G. T., SHAPSHAY, S. M.: Treatment of upper aerodigestive tract cancers with the CO_2 laser. ENT J. **61**, 507 (1982)

DAVIS, K. R., SHAPSHAY, S. M., STRONG, S. M., HYAMS, V. J.: Transoral partial supraglottic resection using the CO_2 laser. Laryngoscope **93**, 429 (1983)

DEDO, H. H., JACKLER, R. K.: Laryngeal papilloma: Results of treatment with the CO_2 laser and podophyllum. Ann. Otol. Rhinol Laryngol. **91**, 425 (1982)

DEDO, H. H., SOOY, C. D.: Endoscopic laser repair of posterior glottic, subglottic and tracheal stenosis by division or micro-trapdoor flap. Laryngoscope **94**, 445 (1984)

DI BARTOLOMEO, J. R.: Laser is modern otolaryngology. Trans. Pac. Coart. Otoophthalmol. Soc. **60**, 65 (1979)

DI BARTOLOMEO, J. R., ELLIS, M.: The argon laser in otology. Laryngoscope **90**, 1786 (1980)

DI BARTOLOMEO, J. R.: The argon and CO_2 lasers in otolaryngology: which one, when and why? Laryngoscope 1981 Suppl. 26

DINSTL, K., FISCHER, P. L.: Der Laser. Berlin-Heidelberg-New York, Springer (1981)

DONNADIEU, S., CHANU, D., MILLER, B., BRASNU, D., LACAU-SAINT-GUILY, J.: Critères de choix d'une technique anestésique pour la micro-chirurgie laryngée au laser de l'adulte. Ann. Oto-Laryng. (Paris) **100**, 383 (1983)

DUNCAVAGE, J. A., OSSOFF, R. H., TOOHILL, R. J.: Carbon dioxide laser management of laryngeal stenosis. Ann. otol. (St. Louis) **94**, 565 (1985)

EDELIST, G., ALBERT, P. W.: Anesthesia for CO_2 laser surgery of the larynx. J. Otolaryng. **11**, 107 (1982)

EHRENBERGER, K., INNITZER, J.: Die Wirkung des CO_2-Lasers auf Hautlymphgefäße. Klin. Wschr. (Wien) **90**, 307 (1978)

EICHLER, J. J., KNOF, H., SALK, G., SCHAFER, G., LENZ, H.: Ein Laser-Endoskop für Nasenhaupthöhle, Epipharynx und Kieferhöhle. HNO (Berl.) **26**, 213 (1978)

ESCUDERO, L. H., CASTRO, A. O., DRUMOND, M., PORTO, S. P., BOZINIS, D. G., PENNA, F. S., GALLEGO-LLUSEMA, E.: Argon laser in human tympanoplasty. Arch. Otolaryngol. **105**, 252 (1979)

ESKEW, J. R., BAILEY, B. J.: Laser aryteoidectomy for bilateral vocal cord paralysis. Otol. Head Neck Surg. **91**, 294 (1983)

ÉLŐ, J., REJTŐ, K., POLONY, I., REMENÁR, É., BACSA, L.: Nem-malignus gégeelváltozások laser therápiája. Orv. Hetil. **124**, 1629 (1983)

FANKHAUSER, F.: Der heutige Stand der Laserchirurgie. Schweiz. med. Wschr. **101**, 1425 (1971)

FEDER, R. J.: Laryngeal granuloma as a complication of the CO_2 laser. Laryngoscope **93**, 944 (1983)

FELDMAN, M., UCMAKLI, A., STRONG, S., BAUGHAN, CH., KIM, S., BYLINSKI, A.: Applications of carbon dioxide laser surgery and radiation. Arch. Otolaryngol. **109**, 240 (1983)

FIDLER, J. P., LAW, E., ROCKWELL, R. J., MACMILLAN, B. G.: Carbon dioxide laser excision of acute burns with immediate autografting. J. Surg. Res. **17**, 1 (1974a)

FIDLER, J. P., ROCKWELL, R. J., SILER, V. E., MACMILLAN, B. G., ALTEMEIER, W. A.: Early laser excision of thermal burns in the white rat and miniature pig. Burns. **1**, 5 (1974b)

FIDLER, J. P., LAW, E., ROCKWELL, R. J., MACMILLAN, B. G.: Carbon dioxide laser excision of acute burns with immediate autografting. J. Surg. Res. **17**, 1 (1974)

FIDLER, J. P., HOEFFER, R. W., POLANYI, T. G., BREDEMIER, H. C., SILLER, V. E., ALTEMEIER, W. A.: Laser surgery in exsanguinating liver injury. Ann. Surg. **181**, 74 (1975a)

FIDLER, J. P., LAW, E., MACMILLAN, B. G., FOX, S. G., ROCKWELL, R. J.: Comparison of carbon dioxide laser excision of burns with other thermal knives. Ann. NY. Acad. Sci. **267**, 254 (1975b)

FIDLER, J. P., HOEFFER, R. W., POLANYI, P. E.,BREDEMIER, H. C., SILLER, V. E., ALTEMEIER, W. A.: Laser surgery in exsanguinated liver injury. Am Surg **181**, 74 (1975c)

FISCHER, P. L., DINSTL, K.: Experimentelle Untersuchungen zur Ignitionsgefahr von Tuben bei endolaryngealer Mikrochirurgie mit dem Laser. HNO **33**, 134 (1985)

FISCHER, S. E., FRAME, J. W.: The effects of the carbon dioxide surgical laser on oral tissues. Brit. J. oral maxillofac Surg. **22**, 414 (1984)

FRAME, J. W.: Removal of soft tissue pathology with the CO_2 laser. J. oral maxillofac Surg. **43**, 850 (1985)

FRIED, M. P.: Complications of CO_2 laser surgery of the larynx. Laryngoscope **93**, 275 (1983)

FRIED, M. P.: Limitations of laser laryngoscopy. Otolaryng. Clin. N. Amer. **17**, 199 (1984)

FRIEDMAN, E. W.: The CO_2 laser in head and neck surgery. Jerusalem Acad. Press. Jesus 63 (1976)

FRIEDMAN, E. W.: The CO_2 laser in head and neck surgery. Jerusalem Acad. Press. Jesus 159 (1978)

FRIEDMAN, E. W., HEALY, G. B., MCGILL, T. J. I.: Carbon dioxide laser management of subglottic and tracheal stenosis. Otolaryng. Clin. N. Amer. **16**, 871 (1983)

FRISHMAN, A., GASSNER, S., KAPLAN, I., GER, R.: Excision of subcutaneous fibrosarcoma in mice. Isr. J. Med. Sci. **10**, 637 (1974)

FUKUTAKE, T., YAMASHITA, T., TOMODA, K., KUMAZAWA, T.: Laser surgery for allergic rhinitis. Arch. Otolaryngol. Head Neck Surg. **112**, 1280 (1986)

GAILLARD, J., HAGUENAUER, J. P., DUBREUIL, C.: Tuilité du laser dans les stenoses laryngo-trachéales acquises et dans les diplégies laryngées. J. Franc. ORL (Lyon) **31**, 261 (1982)

GAILLARD, J., HAGUENAUER, J. P., PIGNAT, J. C., MACHALY, M.: L'utilisation du laser Y.A.G. en O.R.L. (á propos de 147 applications). Cah. O.R.L. Chir.-cervico-fac. **20**, 128 (1985)

GANTZ, B. J., KISHIMOTO, S., JENKINS, H. A., FISCH, U.: Argon laser stapedotomy. Ann. Otol. **91**, 25 (1982)

GILLIS, T. M., STRONG, M. S.: Surgical lasers and soft tissue interactions. Otolaryng. Clin. N. Amer. **16**, 775 (1983)

GLOVER, J. L., BENDICK, P. J., LINK, W. J.: The use of thermal knives in surgery: Electrosurgery, lasers, plasma scalpel. Curr. Probl. Surg. **15**, 1 (1978)

GOFORTH, A. J., COOKE, J. E., PUTNEY, J. F.: An anesthesia technique for laser surgery of the larynx. Laryngoscope **93**, 822 (1983)

GOLDMAN, L.: The biomedical laser. New York-Heidelberg-Berlin, Springer (1981)

GROSSENBACHER, R.: Erfahrungen mit der CO_2-Laserchirurgie in der Otorhinolaryngologie. HNO **27**, 403 (1979)

GROSSENBACHER, R.: Der CO_2-Laser in der Hals-Nasen-Ohren-Chirurgie. Schweiz. med. Wschr. **110**, 790 (1980)

GROSSENBACHER, R.: Laserchirurgie in der Oto-Rhino Larygologie. Stuttgart, New York: Georg Thieme (1985)

GROTELÜSCHEN, B.: Der heutige Stand der Chirurgie mit Laserstrahlen. Chirurg **49**, 197 (1978)

GROTELÜSCHEN, B., BUCHOLZ, J.: Untersuchungen zur Schnittcharakteristik beim Schneiden mit Laserstrahlen. 119. Tagung der Vereinigung Nordwestdeutscher Chirurgen, Lübeck, 2.–4. Juni, 1976. In: Zentralbl. Chir. **103**, 385 (1977)

GÜLZOW, J. et al.: Experimentelle Stapesplastik mit den CO_2-Laser. Laryng. Rhinol (Stuttg.) **65**, 208 (1986)

GÜLZOW, J., LENARZ, T.: Stapesplastik mit dem CO_2-Laser am Hund. Zentralbl. 000498

HAGUENAUER, J. P., GAILLARD, J.: L'utilisation du laser en oto-rhino-laryngologie. Revue de LOR (Bordeaux) **102**, 495 (1981)

HALL, R. R., BEACH, A. D., BAKER, E., MORRISON, P. C. A.: Incision of tissue by carbon dioxide laser. Nature (Lond.) **232**, 131 (1971)

HEALY, G. B.: Complications of laser surgery. Otolaryng. Clin. N. Amer. **16**, 815 (1983)

HERBERT, J. T., BERLIN, I., EBERLE, R.: Jet ventilation via a copper endotracheal tube for CO_2 laser surgery of the oropharynx. Laryngoscope **95**, 1276 (1985)

HIRSHMAN, C. A., LEON, D., PORCH, D., EVERTS, E., SMITH, J. D.: Improved metal endotracheal tube for laser surgery of the airway. Anesth. Analg. **59**, 789 (1980)

HISHIMOTO, K., ROCKWELL, R. J. Jr., EPSTEIN, R. A., YUNIS, N. G., FIDLER, J. P.: Plasma salpel surgery: report of some experimental evaluations and incidence of gas embolt. Burns. **1**, 128 (1975)

HOBEIKA, C. P., ROCKWELL, R. J.: Argon laser microsurgery: its advantages and applications in otolaryngology. Laryngoscope **83**, 960 (1973)

HOCHLEITNER, F., MEINDL, J.: Der Laser in der Larynxmikrochirurgie – ein Fortschritt. Österr. HNO-Kongr. 1984, 156 (1985)

HOEKSEMA, P. E., OVERBEEK, J. J. M.: CO_2-Laser in microlarynx surgery. ORL (Basel) **40**, 385 (1978)

HOEKSEMA, P. E., OVERBEEK, J. J. M.: Der CO_2-Laser bei Larynxerkrankungen. Acta otorhinolaryng belg. **35**, 23 (1981)

HORCH, H. H.: Laser Osteomie. Habil-Schrift, Düsseldorf (1977)

HOROSZOWSKI, H., FARINE, I., ENGEL, J.: The laser in orthopaedic surgery, in KAPLAN, I. (ed.): Proceedings of the 1st international symposium on laser surgery. Jerusalem, Jerusalem Academic Press, pp **139**, 144 (1976)

HOYE, R. C., MINTON, J. P.: The noble gas laser as a light-knife. Surg Forum **16**, 93 (1965)

HOYE, R. C., WEISS, G. H., KETCHAM, A. S.: Growth rate of experimental tumor after the use of laser energy. J. Nat. Cancer. Inst. **37**, 819 (1966)

HÖFLER, H., BURIAN, K.: Erfahrungen mit der CO_2-Laserchirurgie beim Kehlkopfmalignom und deren funktionelle Ergebnisse. Zentralbl. **127**, 4276 (1981)

HÖFLER, H.: Esperienza sull'-uso del laser in laringologia. Acta ERL Ital. (Pisa) **2**, 107 (1982)

HÖFLER, H.: Ergebnisse der proc. Vocalis-Resection mit dem CO_2-Laser bei beidseitiger Stimmbandlähmung. Zentralbl. **130**, 5539 (1984)

HÖFLER, H.: Langzeitresultate nach CO_2-Laserbehandlung von Larynxkarcinomen. Österr. HNO-Kongr. 1985, 14 (1986)

HUNTON, J., OSWAL, V. H.: Metal tube anaesthesia for ear? Nose and throat carbon dioxide laser surgery. Anaesthesia (Lond.) **40**, 1210 (1985)

INOUYE, T.: Application of CO_2-laser to the carcinoma of the larynx. Auris Nasus Larynx (Tokyo) 12, Suppl. **2**, 178 (1985)

JAKÓ, G. J.: Laser surgery of the vocal cords. An experimental study with carbon dioxide lasers on dogs. Laryngoscope **82**, 2204 (1972)

JAKÓ, G. J.: Microsurgery of the larynx with carbon dioxide laser. Otolaryngology **3**, 1 (1979)

JAKÓ, G. J.: Future directions and developments in laser surgery. Otolaryng. Clin. N. Amer. **16**, 821 (1983)

JAKÓ, G. J.: Microscopic and endocopic laser surgery. Med. Instr. **17**, 407 (1983)

JAKÓ, G. J.: The use of lasers in cancer surgery. Springer 1984 Boston.

JAKÓ, G. J., FABIANI, M.: La chirurgia con in laser CO_2 in otorinolaringoiatria. Riv. ital. ORL Audiol. Foniat. **2**, 343 (1982)

JAKÓ, G. J., POLANYI, T. G.: Carbon dioxide laser surgery in otolaryngology. In: KAPLAN I., p 149

JAKÓ, G. J., POLANYI, T. G.: Carbon dioxide laser surgery in otolaryngology. Jerusalem Acad. Press. Jesus 149 (1976)

JAKÓ, G. J., POLANYI, T. G.: Carbon dioxide laser surgery in otolaryngology. In KAPLAN, I.: Laser surgery. Academic Press, Jerusalem (1976)

JAKÓ, G. J., STRONG, M. S.: Experimental carbon dioxide laser surgery of the vocal cords. Eye Ear Nose Thr. Monthly **52**, 171 (1973)

JAKÓ, G. J., VAUGHAN, CH. W., STRONG, M. S., POLANYI, TH. G.: Surgical management of malignant tumors of the aerodigestive tract with carbon dioxide laser microsurgery. Intern. Adv. Surg. Onc. **1**, 265 (1978)

JANCZEWSKI, G., SONNENBERG, Z., POLUBINSKI, R.: Experimental investigations on the effect of CO_2-laser on living tissue. Preliminary report. Otolaryng. Polsk. **36**, 137 (1982)

JANCZEWSKI, G., SONNENBERG, Z., POLUBINSKI, R.: CO_2-laser as a surgical instrument. Otolaryng. Polsk. **36**, 181 (1982)

JANTZEN, J. P., HILLEY, D.: Ein neuer Tubus für Laser-Eingriffe am Larynx. Anaesthesist **32**, 502 (1983)

JANTZEN, J. P.: Endotrachealtuben für CO_2-Laserchirurgie des Larynx. HNO **32**, 28 (1984)

KAEDER, C. S., HIRSHMAN, C. A.: Acute airway obstruction: A complication of aluminium tape wrapping of tracheal tubes in laser surgery. Canad. Anaesth. Soc. J. **26**, 139 (1979)

KAPLAN, I.: Laser surgery – Proceedings of the 1st International Symposium on Laser Surgery. Israel. Jerusalem Academic Press, Jerusalem (Kl) (1976)

KAPLAN, I., GER, R.: The carbon dioxide laser in clinical surgery: a preliminary report. Israel J. Med. Sci. **9**, 79 (1973)

KAPLAN, I., GER, R.: Partial mastectomy and mammaplasty performed with a CO_2 surgical laser: a comparative study. Brit. J. Plast. Surg. **26**, 363 (1973)

KARDUCK, A., RICHTER, H. G.: Laser-Chirurgie des Stimmbandes. Tierexperimentelle Untersuchungen. Laryng. Rhinol. **55**, 144 (1976)

KARDUCK, A., RICHTER, H. G.: Experimental studies on neodym-YAG-laser microsurgery of the vocal cords in dogs. Acta oto-rhino-laryng. belg. **31**, 81 (1977)

KARDUCK, A., RICHTER, H. G., BLANK, M.: Laserchirurgie des Stimmbandes. Laryng. Rhinol. **57**, 419 (1978)

KARDUCK, A., BLANK, M.: Was kann von der endolaryngealen Anwendung des neodym-YAG-Lasers als Behandlungsmethode erwartet werden? HNO **27**, 298 (1979)

KARDUCK, A., RICHTER, H. G.: Lasermikrochirurgische Behandlung gutartiger Stimmlippenveränderungen und ihre funktionellen Ergebnisse. Laryng. Rhinol. **58**, 764 (1979)

KÁSLER, M., PÓLUS, K., BÁNHIDY, F., VESZPRÉMI, Z., ZEMPLÉN, B.: Probleme der akuten Tracheotomie mittels CO_2-Laser bei extrem großen Schilddrüsenkrebsen. Wiss. Zeitschr. **33**, 187 (1984)

KOUFMAN, J. A., THOMPSON, J. N., KOHUT, R. I.: Endoscopic management of subglottic stenosis with the CO_2 surgical laser. Otolaryng. Head Neck Surg. **89**, 215 (1981)

KRAJINA, Z.: Esperienza sull'uso del laser in laringologia. Acta ORL ital. (Pisa) **2**, 99 (1982)

KRÉMER, I., MÉSZÁROS, I., BOROSS, J., BÁNHIDY, F., KÁSLER, M.: Az endolaryngeális laser műtétek anaesthesiája. Anaesthesiológiai és Intenziv Therapia, **13**, 61 (1983)

KUMAR, A., FROST, E.: Anesthesiology **54**, 350 (1981)

KÜTTNER, J., ALBEGGER, K.: Brandgefahr bei endolyrangealer Laserchirurgie. Österr. HNO-Kongr. 1984, 168 (1985)

LACCOURREYE, H., LACAU SAINT-GUILY, J., BRASNU, D., DONNADIEU, S., POPOT, B., GUTTON, O., PARPOUNAS, C.: Utilisation du laser CO_2 dans le traitment d'urgence des dyspnées des cancers du larynx. Ann. Oto-Laryng. (Paris), **101**, 39 (1984)

LANG, G. F.: Laserchirurgie – eine neue Operationsmethode. HNO **31**, 349 (1983)

LEJEUNE, F. E., GUICE, C., LETARD, F., MARICE, H.: Heat sink protection against lasering endotracheal cuffs. Ann. ORL **91**, 606 (1982)

LENZ, H., WULLSTEIN, H. K., EICHLER, J.: Morphologische Veränderungen der Schleimhaut nach Bestrahlung mit einem Argonlaser. Eine Tierexperimentelle Studie. Laryng. Rhinol. **55**, 794 (1976)

LENZ, H., EICHLER, J., KNOF, J., SALK, J., SCHÄFER, G.: Endonasales Ar^+-Laser-Strahlführungssystem und erste klinische Anwendungen bei der Rhinopathia Vasomotorica. Laryng. Rhinol. **56**, 749 (1977)

LENZ, H.: Tonsillektomie mit einem Laserraspatorium. Laryng. Rhinol. Otol. **63**, 582 (1984)

LENZ, H.: Acht Jahre Laserchirurgie an den unteren Nasenmuscheln bei Rhinopathia Vasomotorica in Form der Laserstrichkarbonisation. HNO **33**, 422 (1985)

LEVINE, N., SEIFTER, E., GER, R., STELLAR, S., LEVENSON, S. M.: Use of carbon-dioxide laser for the debridement of third degree burns. Abstract book, Fourth Annual Meeting. American Burn Association, San Francisco (1972)

LEVINE, N. S., SALISBURY, R. E., PATERSON, H. D., PRUITT, B. A.: Clinical evaluation of the carbon dioxide laser for burn wound excisions: a comparison of the laser? Scalpel and electrocautery. J. Trauma **15**, 800 (1975)

LIM, R. Y.: Laser arytenoidectomy. Arch. Otolaryng. (Chicago) **111**, 262 (1985)

LIMA, J. A., WILPIZESKI, CH. R.: Effectiveness of the CO_2 laser in experimental tympanic neurectomy. Laryngoscope **90**, 414 (1980)

LYONS, G. D., LOUSTEAU, R. J., MOUNEY, D. F.: CO_2 laser laryngoscopy in a variety of lesions. Laryngoscope **86**, 1658 (1976)

LYONS, G. D., LOUSTEAU, R. J., MOUNEY, D. F.: CO_2 laser as a clinical tool in otolaryngology. Laryngoscope **87**, 689 (1977)

LYONS, G. D., SCHLOSSER, J. V., LOUSTEAU, R., MOUNEY, D. F., BENES, E. N.: Laser surgery and immunotherapy in the management of laryngeal papilloma. Laryngoscope **88**, 1586 (1978)

LYONS, G. D., OWENS, R., LOUSTEAU, R. J., TRALL, M. L.: Carbon dioxide laser treatment of laryngeal stenosis. Arch. Otolaryngol (Chicago) **106**, 255 (1980)

LYONS, G. D., LOUSTEAU, R. J.: CO_2 laser management of laryngeal stenosis. ENT J. **61**, 505 (1982)

MCGEE, K. C., NAGLE, J. W., TOOHIL, R. J.: CO_2 laser repair of subglottic and upper tracheal stenosis: Otolaryngology (Rochester, MN) **89**, 92 (1981)

McGee, T. M.: The argon laser in surgery for chronic ear disease and otosclerosis. Laryngoscope **93**, 1177 (1983)

McGuff, P. E., Deterling, R. A., Gottlieb, L. S., Fapimi, H. D., Bushnell, D.: Surgical applications of lasers. Ann. Surg. **160**, 765 (1964)

MacMillan, B. G.: Closing the burn wound. Surg. Clin. NA **58**, 1205 (1978)

Madden, J. E., Edlich, R. F., Cuater, J. R., Rauck, P. H., Therl, J., Wagensteen, O. H.: Studies in the management of the contaminated wound. IV. Resistance to infection of surgical wounds made by knife, electrosurgery, and laser. Am. J. Surg. **119**, 222 (1970)

Matthias, R., Schüssler, U., Handrock, M.: Die Innenohrfunktion nach Laser-Stapedotomie. Eine tierexperimentelle Studie. Zentralbl. **129**, 7, 697

Mester, E., Szende, B., Tota, J. G.: Die Wirkung der über längere Zeit wiederholt verabreichten Laserstrahlung geringer Intensität auf die Haut und inneren Organe von Mäusen. Rad. biol. Ther. **10**, 371 (1969)

Meyers, A.: Complications of CO_2 laser surgery of the larynx. Ann. Otol. **90**, 132 (1981)

Miehlke, A., Chilla, R., Vollrath, M.: Cryosurgery and laser surgery in the treatment of malignant and benign laryngeal processes. ORL (Basel) **41**, 263 (1979)

Miehlke, A., Vollrath, M.: Mikroskopische Laser-Chirurgie im Kehlkopfbereich. Dt. Ärzteblatt **4**, 177 (1980)

Miehlke, A., Chilla, R., Vollrath, M.: Die Kryo- und Laserchirurgie zur Behandlung maligner und benigner Kehlkopfprozesse. HNO **28**, 357 (1980)

Mihashi, S., Jakó, G. J., Incze, J. et al.: Laser surgery in otolaryngology: Interaction of CO_2 laser and soft tissue. Ann. Acad. Sci. **267**, 263 (1976)

Miller, D. W., Geraci, J. L., Shumrick, D. A.: Smoke evacuater for laser surgery. Otolaryng. Head Neck Surg. **91**, 582 (1983)

Moore, J. H.: Laser energy in orthopedic surgery. International congress of orthopedic surgeons. Tel-Aviv (1972)

Morgan, A.: Uso del laser in laringologia pediatrica. Acta ORL ital. **2**, 121 (1982)

Morgan, A. H., Norris, J. W., Hicks, J. N.: Palliative laser surgery for melanoma metastatic to the larynx: Report of two cases. Laryngoscope **95**, 794 (1985)

Morscher, E., Rittmann, W. W., Marbet, G. A. et al.: Die Anwendung von Laserstrahlen bei Operationen an Hämophilen. Therapeut Umschau **36**, 316 (1979)

Motta, G., Villari, G., Motta, G. Jr., Ripa, G., Salerno, G.: The CO_2 laser in the laryngeal microsurgery. Acta Otolaryng. (Stockholm) Suppl. 433 (1986)

Muler, H., Prache, H., Marfel, Cl., Seiter, P., Benzekri, P.: Papillomatose profonde de l'adulte et laser. Ann. Oto-laryng. (Paris) **98**, 125 (1981)

Muler, H., Monet, A., Prache, H., Bancel, C., Setier, P.: Laser et phonochirurgie. Ann. Oto-laryng. (Paris) **98**, 129 (1981)

Muler, H., Peytral, Cl., Prache, H., Loubi, G., Setier, P.: Étud expérimentale de la profondeur du rayon laser sur le larynx. Ann Oto-laryng. (Paris) **98**, 141 (1981)

Muler, H., Prache, H., Mardel, C., Bancel, C., Emile, F.: Comparaison des résultats obtenus par le laser et l'instrumentation conventionelle en phonochirurgie. Ann. Oto-laryng. (Paris) **101**, 407 (1984)

Muler, H., Pextral, C., Vacher, S., Henin, J. M., Mak, D., Aubert, Ph.: Bilan de six années de microchirurgie au laser CO_2 en Laryngologie. Ann. Oto-laryng. (Paris) **101**, 411 (1984)

Mullins, F., Jennings, B., McClusky, L.: Liver resections with the continuous wave carbon dioxide laser: Some experimental observations. Amer. Surg. **34**, 717 (1968)

Németh, G., Bánhidy, F.: Telekobalt besugárzás a gégekarcinoma CO_2 lézeres kezelése után. Fül-orr-gégegyógy **31**, 176 (1985)

Norris, C. W., Mullarky, M. B.: Experimental skin incision made with the carbon dioxide laser. Laryngoscope **92**, 416 (1982)

Norton, M. L., Strong, M. S., Vaughan, Ch. W., Snow, J. C., Kripke, B. J.: Endotracheal intubation and venturi (jet) ventilation for laser microsurgery of the larynx. Ann. Otol. (St. Louis) **85**, 656 (1976)

NORTON, M. L., VOS, P.: Endotracheal tube for laser surgery of the larynx. Ann. Otol. (St. Louis) 87, 554 (1978)

NORTON, H. L., DEVOS, P.: New endotracheal tube for laser surgery of the larynx and trachea. Anesthesia **53**, 507 (1979)

OOSTERHUIS, J. W., VERSCHUEREN, R. C. J., OLDHOFF, J.: Experimental surgery on the Cloudman S91 melanoma with the carbon-dioxide laser. Acta Chir. Belg. **74**, 422 (1975)

OOSTERHUIS, J. W.: Tumor surgery with the CO_2 laser: studies with the Cloudman S91 mouse melanoma. PhD Thesis-State University, Groningen, The Netherland (1977)

OSSOFF, R. H., KARLAN, R. H., SISSON, G. A.: Posterior commissure laryngoscope for carbon dioxide laser surgery. Ann. Otol. (St. Louis) **92**, 361 (1983)

OSSOFF, R. H., HOTALING, A. J., KARLAN, M. S., SISSON, G. A.: CO_2 laser in otolaryngology-head and neck surgery: a retrospective analysis of complications. Laryngoscope **93**, 1287 (1983)

OSSOFF, R. H., SISSON, G. A., DUNCAVAGE, J. A., MOSELLE, H. I., ANDREWS, PH. E., MCMILLAN, W. G.: Endoscopic laser arytenoidectomy for the treatment of bilateral vocal cord paralysis. Laryngoscope **94**, 1293 (1984)

PATEL, C. K. N., TIEN, P. K., MCFEE, J. H.: CW High-power CO_2-N_2-HE laser. Appl. Phys. Lett. **7**, 290 (1965)

PATIL, V., STEHLING, L. C., ZAUDER, H. L.: A modified endotracheal tube for laser microsurgery. Anesthesiology **51**, 571 (1979)

PELED, I., SHOHAT, B., GASSNER, S., KAPLAN, I.: Excision of eptihelial tumors: CO_2 laser versus conventional methods. Cancer Letters **2**, 41 (1976)

PERKINS, R. C.: Laser stapedotomy for otosclerosis. Laryngoscope **90**, 228 (1980)

PERRIN, C.: Revue des indications de la chirurgie laser en ORL. (á propos de 110 cas) J. Franc. ORL **30**, 657 (1981)

PEYTRAL, C., VACHER, S., AUBERT, PH., MULER, H.: Repermeabilisation de la filière laryngèe par le laser. Ann. Oto-laryng. (Paris) **101**, 415 (1984)

PIGNAL, C., GUETAT, M., PIGNAT, J., GAILLARD, J., DUBREULL, C.: Anesthèsie pour laser en ORL sans intubation à propos de 961 cas personnels. J. Franc. ORL **31**, 643 (1982)

PIQUET, J. J., DARRAS, J. A., BUISSET, E.: Le traitement au laser CO_2 des laryngo-pyocelès. J. Franc. ORL **31**, 716 (1982)

PIQUET, J. J., DARRAS, J. A., BURNY, A., TON, VAN, J., VERPLANKEN, M.: Le traitement endoscopique au laser des kystes du larynx et des laryngocèles. Ann. Oto laryng (Paris) **101**, 283 (1984)

PRAMESBERGER, G., FISCHER, P. L., BENKE, A., GLANINGER, J.: Experiences with a non-inflammable tube for laser surgery of the larynx. Anaesthesist **34**, 636 (1985)

PRASAD, U.: CO_2 surgical laser in the management of bilateral vocal cord paralysis. J. Laryng. Otol. **99**, 891 (1985)

REMSEN, K., LAWSON, W., PATEL, N., BILLER, H. F.: Laser lateralization for bilateral vocal cord abductor paralysis. Otolaryng Head Neck Surg **93**, 645 (1985)

RICHTER, H. G., SCHUCHARDT, W.: Messungen der Wärmeleitung unterschiedlicher Gewebe und ihre Bedeutung für die Laserchirurgie des Larynx. HNO **29**, 163 (1981)

RIBÁRI, O., JÓRI, J., KISS, G., VÓNA, I., TOMITY, I.: Forderung des Verschlusses von künstlichen Trommelfellperforationen mit energiearmer He-Ne-Laserbestrahlung. Acta Chir. Acad. Scint. Hung. **21**, 229 (1980)

RIBÁRI, O.: The stimulating effect of low power laser rays: experimental examinations in otolaryngology. Rev. Laryng. (Bordeaux) **102**, 531 (1981)

RONTAL, M., RONTAL, E.: Treatment of recurrent carcinoma at the base of the skull with carbon dioxide laser. Laryngoscope **93**, 1261 (1983)

RONTAL, E., RONTAL, M., WENOKUR, M. E.: Jet insufflation anesthesia for endolaryngeal laser surgery: A review of 318 consecutive cases. Laryngoscope **95**, 990 (1985)

ROUNDS, D. E., OLSEN, R. S., BOUHER, J.: Measurements of the cell migration index with a He Ne laser. Ann. NY Acad. Sci. **26**, 152 (1979)

RUDERTH, H.: Erfahrungen mit dem CO_2-Laser unter besonderer Berücksichtigung der Therapie von Stimmbandkarzinomen. Laryng. Rhinol. Otol. **62**, 493 (1983)

RUOPPOLO, G. et al.: L'utilissazione del laser CO_2 nella microchirurgia laringea. Il Valsalva (Roma) **61**, 237 (1985).

SAKS, N. M., ROTH, C. A.: Die Ultrastruktur von Haut- und Schleimhautgeweben nach CO_2-Lasereinwirkung. Laryng. Rhinol. **58**, 770 (1979)

SCHRAMM, V. L., MATTOX, D. E., STOOL, S. E.: Acute management of laser-ignited intratracheal explosion. Laryngoscope **91**, 1417 (1981)

SHAKER, M. H., KONCHIGERI, H. N., ANDREWS, A. H., HOLINGER, P. H.: Anesthetic management for carbon dioxide laser surgery of the larynx. Laryngoscope **86**, 857 (1976)

SHAPSHAY, ST. M.: Use of the CO_2 laser in diagnosis and staging. Head and Neck Cancer J. Wiley Sons New York 1986

SHUGAR, J. M., SOM, P. M., BILLER, H. F.: An evaluation of the carbon dioxide laser in the treatment of traumatic laryngeal stenosis. Laryngoscope **92**, 23 (1982)

SIMPSON, G. T., HEALY, G. B., MCGILL, T., STRONG, M. S.: Benign tumors and lesions of the larynx in children: surgical excision by CO_2 laser. Ann Otol. **88**, 479 (1979)

SIMPSON, G. T., SHAPSHAY, S. M., VAUGHN, CH. W., STRONG, S. M.: Rhinologic sugery with the carbon dioxide laser. Laryngoscope **92**, 412 (1982)

SIMPSON, G. T., POLANYI, T. G.: History of the carbon dioxide laser in otolaryngologic surgery. Otolaryng. Clin. N. Amer. **16**, 739 (1983)

SIMPSON, G. T., STRONG, M. S.: Recurrent respiratory papillomatosis: the role of the carbon dioxide laser. Otolaryng. Clin. N. Amer. **16**, 887 (1983)

SNOW, J. C., KRIPKE, B. J., STRONG, M. S., JAKÓ, G. J., MEYER, M. R., VAUGHAN, CH. W.: Anesthesia for carbon dioxide laser microsurgery on the larynx and trachea. Anesth. Analg. **53**, 507 (1974)

SNOW, J. C., NORTON, M. L., SALUJA, T. S., ESTANISLAO, A. F.: Fire hazard during to CO_2 laser microsurgery on the larynx and trachea. Anesth. Analg. **55**, 146 (1976)

SORENSEN, H.: Laser surgery in benignant laryngeal disease. Acta Otolaryngol. Suppl. **386**, 177 (1982)

SORENSEN, H.: Laser surgery in benign laryngeal disease. Acta Otolaryngol. **94**, 537 (1982)

SÖDERBERG, O. et al.: Uyzingotomy made by CO_2 laser. Au alternative to the ventilation tube? An experimental study. Acta Oto-laryng. (Stockholm) **97**, 335 (1984)

SCHLOSSHAUER, B., STÄDTLER, F.: Grenzen der endolaryngealen CO_2-Laserchirurgie des Stummlippenkarzinoms. HNO **30**, 293 (1982)

STEINER, W.: Esperienza sull'uso del laser in laryngologia. Acta ORL ital. **2**, 113 (1982)

STELLAR, S., MEIJER, R., WALLA, S., et al.: Carbon dioxide laser debridement of decubitus uclers: followed by immediate rotation flap or skingraft closure. Ann. Surg. **179**, 230 (1974)

STELLAR, S., POLANYI, T. E., BREDEMEIER, H. C.: Lasers in surgery. In: Laser application in medicine and biology. Vol 2 Pleuum Press, New York, p **241**, 293 (1974)

STERN, L. S., ABRAMSON, A. L., GRIMES, G. W.: Qualitative and morphometric evaluation of vocal cord lesions produced by the carbon dioxide laser. Laryngoscope **90**, 792 (1980)

STRONG, M. S.: Laser management of premalignant lesions of the larynx. Canad. J. Otolaryng. **3**, 560 (1974)

STRONG, M. S.: Laser excision of carcinoma of the larynx. Laryngoscope **85**, 1286 (1975)

STRONG, M. S., JAKÓ, G. J.: Laser surgery in the larynx; early clinical experience with continuous CO_2 laser. Ann. Otol. (St. Louis) **81**, 791 (1982)

STRONG, M. S., JAKÓ, G. J., POLANYI, T. G., WALLACE, R. A.: Laser surgery in the aero-digestive tract. Am. J. Surg. **126**, 529 (1973)

STRONG, S. M., JAKÓ, G. J., VAUGHAN, CH. W., HEALY, G. B., POLANYI, TH.: The use of the CO_2 laser in otolaryngology: a progress report. Trans Amer. Acad. Ophthal. Otolaryng. **82**, 595 (1976)

STRONG, M. S., VAUGHAN, CH. W., HEALY, G. B., COOPERBAND, S. R., CLEMENT, M. A.: Recurrent respiratory papillomatosis: management with the CO_2 laser. Ann. Otol. (St. Louis) **85**, 508 (1976)

STRONG, M. S., VAUGHAN, C. W., HEALY, G. B.: Recurrent respiratory papillomatosis in laryngotracheal problems in pediatric patients. In HEALY, G. B., MCGILL, T. (eds.): Textbooks of ear, nose, throat. Springfield, III, Charles C Thomas, pp **88**, 98 (1979)

THOMA, J. et al.: Experimental investigations on the suitability of the carbon dioxide laser for stapendotomy. Ann. Otolaryng. (St. Louis) **95**, 126 (1986)

TICHY, S.: CO_2-Laser-Therapie von Kehlkopfstenosen. Wiss. Zeitschr. **33**, 244 (1984)

TIMEN, G. R., VINNICHUK, P. V.: Laser therapy in patients with nasal furuncle. Z usn nos gorlov Bolezn 3, 6 (1986)

TIMIGRALEEV, M. K., SHUSTER, M. A., GAVRILENKO, S. L.: Transtubal laser radiation therapy of inflammatory diseases of the auditory tube and the middle ear. Vestn. ORL (Mosk.) **1**, 63 (1986)

TRANTER, R. M. D., PLATT, S. E., FRANE, J. W. et al.: A comparative study of the healing of lasered and surgically excised wounds in the upper aerodigestive tract. Clin. Otolaryng. **7**, 283 (1982)

VAUGHAN, CH. W.: Transoral laryngeal surgery using the CO_2 laser: Laboratory experiments and clinical experience. Laryngoscope **88**, 1399 (1978)

VAUGHAN, CH. W., STRONG, M. S., JAKÓ, G. J.: Laryngeal carcinoma: transoral treatment utilizing the CO_2 laser. Amer. J. Surg. **136**, 490 (1978)

VAUGHAN, C. W.: Use of the carbon dioxide laser in the endoscopic management of organic laryngeal disease. Otolaryng. Clin. N. Amer. **16**, 849 (1983)

VECERINA, S., KRAJINA, Z.: Phonotory function following unilateral laser cordectomy. J. Laryng. **97**, 1139 (1983)

VERHULST, J., VERHULST, D.: Le laser en O.R.L. Rev. Laryng. (Bordeaux) **100**, 247 (1979)

VERSCHUEREN, R.: The CO_2 laser in tumor surgery. Amsterdam, Van Gorcum, (Assen), (1976)

VOLLRATH, M., RALPH, G.: Lichtmikroskopische und elektronenoptische Befunde bei CO_2-Laser-induzierten Gefäßveränderungen. HNO **29**, 153 (1981)

VOLLRATH, R., RALPH, G.: Gefäßveränderungen durch den CO_2-Laser. HNO **29**, 249 (1981)

VOLLRATH, M., SCHREINER, C.: Influence of argon laser stapedotomy on inner ear function and temperature. Otolaryng. Head Neck Surg. **91**, 521 (1983)

VOLLRATH, M., SCHREINER, CHR.: Influence of argon laser stapedotomy on cochlear potentials. Acta Otolaryngol **96**, 49 (1983)

WEERDA, H., PEDERSEN, P., WEHMER, H., BRAUNE, H.: Ein neues Laryngoskop für die endolaryngeale Mikrochirurgie. Arch. Otorhinolaryngol. **225**, 103 (1979)

WETMORE, S. J., KEY, M. J., SUEN, J. Y.: Complications of laser surgery for laryngeal papillomatosis. Laryngoscope **95**, 798 (1985)

WETMORE, S. J., KEY, M. J., SUEN, J. Y.: Laser therapy for T_1 glottic carcinoma of the larynx. Arch. Otolaryngol **112**, 853 (1986)

WILLIAMS, D. J., HUNTER-DUVAR, I. M., MITCHELL, D. P.: Use of the CO_2 laser in otology. Ann. Otolaryng. (St. Louis) **90**, 70 (1981)

WOO, P., VAUGHAN, C. W.: A safe, nonflammable, all-metal, cuffless endotracheal venturi ventilation system for use in laser surgery. Otolaryng. Head Neck Surg. **91**, 497 (1983)

YARINGTON, C. T., THOMPSON, G. E.: Incendiary characteristics and endotracheal tubes with one carbon dioxide laser. Ann. Otol. (St. Louis) **91**, 605 (1982)

YATES, A., DEDO, H. H.: Carbon dioxide laser enucleation of polypoid vocal cords. Laryngoscope **94**, 731 (1984)

YOUNG, R. J.: Laser surgery for T_1 glottic carcinoma – The argument against. J. Laryng. (London) **97**, 243 (1983)

MIX
Papier | Fördert gute Waldnutzung
FSC® C083411

Zeitfracht Medien GmbH
Ferdinand-Jühlke-Straße 7
99095 Erfurt, Deutschland
produktsicherheit@kolibri360.de